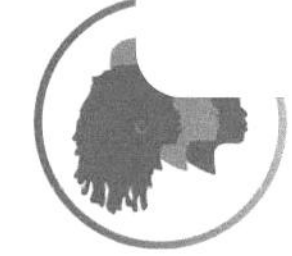

Healing

IN REVIEW

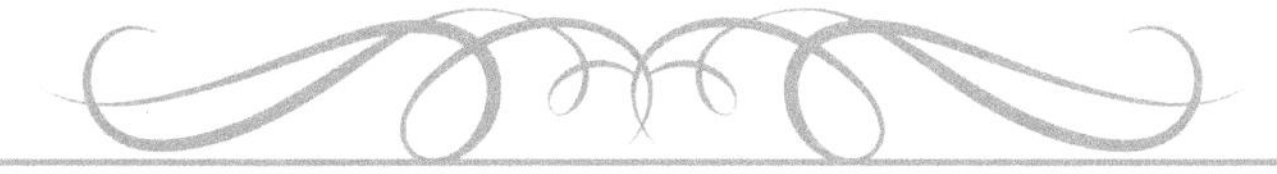

A guide for those seeking or already in counseling or coaching. Tools and resources on finding a coach or counselor, along with guided reflections on preparing for your sessions and tracking progress.

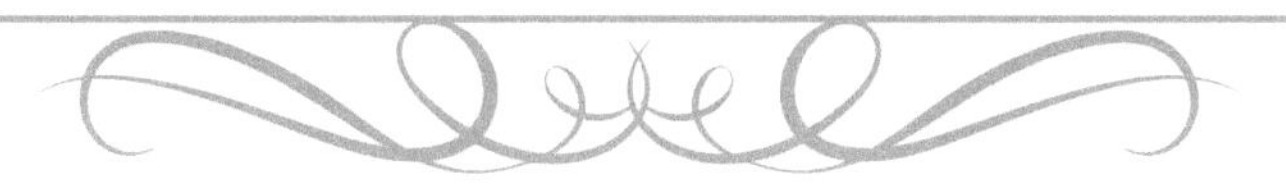

A JOURNEY FROM SURVIVING TO THRIVING

by Dr. Sherra' Watkins

Foreword By: Tish Guerin, MSW, LCSW

This is a work of fiction. Names, characters, places, and incidents either are the product of the author's imagination or are used fictitiously. Any resemblance to actual persons, living or dead, events, or locales is entirely coincidental.

Copyright © 2022 by Dr. Sherrá M. Watkins

All rights reserved. No part of this book may be reproduced or used in any manner without written permission of the copyright owner except for the use of quotations in a book review. For more information, address: drsherra@sisterwells.org.

First paperback edition March 2022

Book design by Dr. Sherrá M. Watkins
Sister WELLS Counseling, Coaching & Consulting, PLLC

ISBN 979-8-9855349-0-0 (paperback)
ISBN 979-8-9855349-2-4 (spiral book)

www.sisterwells.org

THIS JOURNAL

BELONGS TO:

IF FOUND, PLEASE RETURN TO:

Table of Contents

NO.	TITLE	PAGE NO.
1.	Book Overview	6
2.	How to Use the Journal	7
3.	Do I Need Counseling/Coaching	8
4.	Wellness Assessment	9
5.	Before You Start	14
6.	Coaching vs. Counseling	15
7.	Finding a Coach or Counselor	18
8.	Appointment Tracker	24
9.	Managing Medications	26
10.	Setting Goals	27
11.	What To Expect	33
12.	Tracking My Healing Process	34
13.	Guided Interventions	172
14.	Resources: Phone Apps	199
15.	Common Terms & Acronyms	201
16.	Acknowledgments	202
17.	About the Author	203

Foreword

Dr. Sherrá Watkins is a dynamic Licensed Psychotherapist who has dedicated her life's work toward ensuring that people have the necessary therapeutic tools to be the best versions of themselves. Her mission to educate on the imperative topics of Mental Health and Substance Abuse, has helped individuals improve overall wellbeing, mend relationships, break generational cycles of trauma, and more importantly, save lives of those fortunate to work with her on their journey to healing.

As a Licensed Psychotherapist myself, I was able to work with Dr. Watkins as she worked tirelessly reinforcing the value of self-care as it relates to clients and patients while also taking time to focus on herself, which can be difficult when you consistently pour into the lives of others. Nevertheless, Dr. Watkins has consistently accomplished this with grace and a keen insight towards making Mental Health and Substance Abuse a staple in the lives of those she touched. While Dr. Watkins and I have different specialties in the field of Mental Health, mine being focused on Athlete Mental Health and Wellness and Dr. Watkins diverse experience in settings of community-based, higher education and hospitals, our purpose is parallel. Mental Health is just as important as physical health. Ensuring that we provide knowledge paired with tangible resources to assist in moving people forward with their Mental Health as a staple in their wellbeing is the mission.

I find solace that Dr. Watkins has chosen to create a valuable tool that will guide individuals on their journey towards healing while simultaneously providing guidance in what to ask, where to go, and what to know for someone seeking support in their Mental Health expedition. As you matriculate through this workbook, you will get all of your questions answered about how to start the conversation towards wholeness. Worksheets, definitions, how to seek a Licensed Therapist, what to ask your Therapist once you have identified them, will all be provided in your exploration through this workbook. Ultimately, this is the book you didn't know you needed. Fortunately, you're here now, and your Mental Health thanks you!

~Tish Guerin, MSW, LCSW, LISW-CP, BC-TMH, CMIP

**Tish Guerin is a Licensed Psychotherapist specializing is Mental Health programming, Certified Mindfulness and Professional Sports Therapy in the United States with Board Certified Licensure in North Carolina, South Carolina, and Pennsylvania.*

INSTAGRAM - https://www.instagram.com/therealdopetherapist

WEBSITE - https://therealdopetherapist.com/

About this Journal

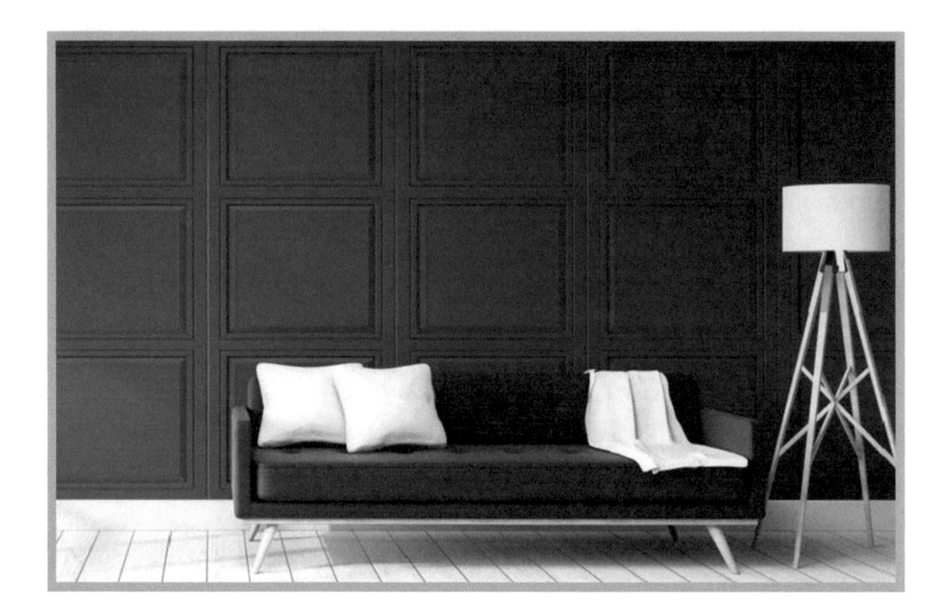

Does it feel like you're losing your true self in the relationship?

Are you struggling to find your purpose?

Have you tried to solve the problems in your life on your own and realized you need help from someone else (Professional help)?

Have you been debating seeking help for weeks, months, or years?

If you answered Yes to any of these questions, then you have made the right choice by being here. You've taken the first step in creating a healthier you. This book was created with you in mind. I have created a comprehensive book that will take you from start to finish with beginning your therapy or coaching process.

Let's get started!

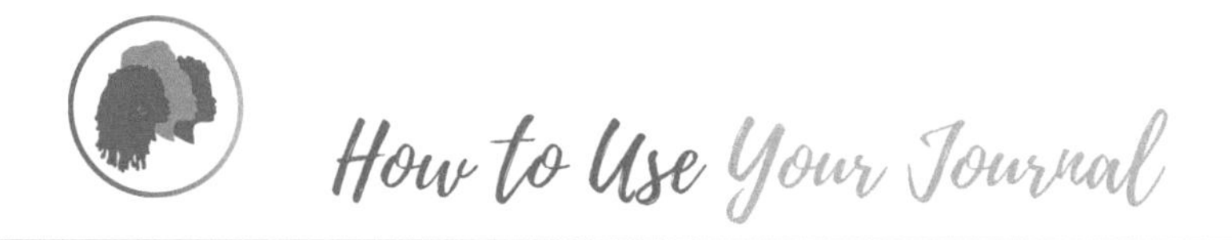

How to Use Your Journal

This journal was designed by a therapist who also benefits from seeking counseling and coaching herself. The journal entries are made to help you track your counseling and coaching sessions, goals, emotions and become more aware of thought patterns, thereby yielding growth.

As a therapist who has utilized both counseling and coaching, I often listened as clients shared their process of finding me and what made them choose me. Some stories are simple as they found me through word of mouth or found me via their insurance or therapy directory, while others shared horror stories of it taking months to find a therapist or horrible experiences with their first experience.

Upon starting services, I watched as some clients also struggled with remembering homework, outcomes of in-session activities, and memorable moments where they were able to "put the pieces of the puzzle together" or 'Aha' moments. Other times, I would watch clients who were just like me struggle to maintain one specific notebook to document their healing process. I would have multiple notebooks or journals with information in each one. As I look back over the years of therapy, there are highlights of significant moments that I vividly remember. However, there were other moments that were just as profound that I could not remember as well, and I wish I had a journal that allowed me to track my progress, symptoms, goals, and even appointments, along with noting highlights from sessions.

Therefore, I created this journal for those who like to journal their thoughts, take notes during and after sessions, and to encourage those who don't to have an easy tool that they can utilize to start the process. I have also provided wellness activities that you can utilize to help towards achieving therapy goals. My hopes are that this journal is more than just a place to jot down information, but a tool that can walk you through the process from start to finish.

WHEN DO I NEED

Counseling or Coaching?

NOTE: Icons listed beside each item denotes which entity (i.e., Coaching or Counseling) would be the best fit to serve that need and/or issue. * Coaching | **Counseling

You're having difficulty regulating your emotions.

We all feel sad, anxious, or angry at some point in our lives. It's important to pay attention to how often or how intensely we feel these emotions.
** / * (depends on the severity)

You want to improve yourself but don't know where to start.

Coaching or counseling can help you identify or become the best version of yourself.
** / * (depends on goals)

You aren't performing as effectively at work or school.

A decrease in performance is a common sign among those struggling with purpose, psychological or emotional issues.
** / * (depends on the severity)

You're Grieving.

Whether it's a divorce, breakup, or loss of a loved one, overcoming grief of any kind can be a long and painful process.**

You're Grieving.

Mental health issues can have a profound impact on our sleep and appetite.
**

You're using alcohol, drugs, or sex to cope.

When you turn to rewarding, numbing, distracting, or destructive things to cope.
** (Counseling Only)

You've experienced trauma.

Those who have a history of physical or sexual abuse or some other trauma that they haven't fully recovered from can also hugely benefit from talk therapy.
** (Counseling Only)

You're struggling to build, maintain or move on from relationships.

People struggling with relationships oftentimes are also struggling with psychological or emotional issues. **

Assessing Your Wellness

Many of us recognize the importance of wellness, but it is easy to get caught up in our busy schedules where we find ourselves not maintaining a holistic regimen that consistently meets our needs. This questionnaire will allow you to determine your level of wellness by rating each of the following dimensions. Although this is not a scientific questionnaire, it will help you become more aware of your current level of wellness and what changes, if any, you might want to make. To complete the questionnaire, please write the number that best describes you.

For each dimension, give yourself:

1 for Rarely, if Ever   2 for Sometimes   3 for Most of the Time   4 for Always

Physical Wellness

1. I maintain my desired weight. ____
2. I engage in vigorous exercise such as brisk walking. ____
3. I do exercise designed to strengthen my muscles and joints. ____
4. I warm-up and cool down by stretching before and after vigorous exercise. ____
5. I feel good about the condition of my body. ____
6. I get 7 – 8 hours of sleep each night. ____
7. My immune system is strong, and I can avoid most infectious diseases. ____
8. My body heals itself quickly when I get sick or injured. ____
9. I have lots of energy and can get through the day without being overly tired. ____
10. I listen to my body; when there is something wrong, I seek professional advice. ____

Social Wellness

1. When I meet people, I feel good about the impression I make on them. ____
2. I am open, honest, and get along well with other people. ____
3. I participate in a wide variety of social activities and enjoy being with people who are different from me. ____
4. I try to be a "better person" and work on behaviors that have caused problems in my interaction with others. ____
5. I get along well with the members of my family. ____
6. I am a good listener. ____
7. I am open and accessible to a loving and responsible relationship. ____
8. I have someone I can talk to about my private feelings. ____
9. I consider the feelings of others and do not act in hurtful or selfish ways. ____
10. I consider how what I say might be perceived by others before I speak. ____

Emotional Wellness

1. I find it easy to laugh about things that happen in my life. ____
2. I avoid using alcohol as a means of helping me forget my problems. ____
3. I can express my feelings without feeling silly. ____
4. When I am angry, I try to let others know in a non-confrontational and non- hurtful way. ____
5. I am not a chronic worrier and tend to be accepting of others. ____
6. I recognize when I am stressed and take steps to relax through exercise, quiet time, or other activities. ____
7. I feel good about myself and believe others like me for who I am. ____
8. When I am upset, I talk to others and actively try to work through my problems. ____
9. I am flexible and adapt or adjust to change in a positive way. ____
10. My friends regard me as a stable, emotionally well-adjusted person. ____

Environmental Wellness

1. I am concerned about environmental pollution and actively try to preserve and protect natural resources. ____
2. I intervene when people intentionally hurt the environment. ____
3. I recycle my garbage. ____
4. I reuse plastic and paper bags and tin foil. ____
5. I vote for pro-environmental candidates in elections. ____
6. I write my elected leaders about environmental concerns. ____
7. I consider the amount of packaging covering a product when I buy my groceries.
8. I try to buy recyclable products. ____
9. I use both sides of the paper when taking class notes or doing assignments. ____
10. I try not to leave the faucet running too long when I brush my teeth, shave or bathe. ____

Spiritual Wellness

1. I believe life is a gift that should be nurtured. ____
2. I take time to enjoy nature and the beauty around me. ____
3. I take time alone to think about what's important in life – who I am, what I value, where I fit in, and where I am going. ____
4. I have consistency between my beliefs, values, and behaviors. ____
5. I engage in acts of caring and goodwill without expecting something in return. ____
6. I feel sorrow for those who are suffering and try to help them through difficult times. ____
7. I feel confident that I have touched the lives of others in a positive way. ____
8. I work for peace in my interpersonal relationship, in my community, and in the world-at-large. ____
9. I am content with who I am. ____
10. I experience life to the fullest. ____

Financial Wellness

1. I have some cash in my possession. ____
2. I check my credit report to look for any errors (TransUnion, Experian, or Equifax). ____
3. I am comfortable with where my money comes from and where it is going. ____
4. I am prepared for sudden financial changes. ____
5. I have a plan in place to pay off debt. ____
6. I use a credit card and am building credit. ____
7. I think about starting a retirement account in the near future. ____
8. I save part of my income in a savings account. ____
9. I am not defined by the amount of money I have in my bank account. ____
10. I review my bank statements when I receive them. ____

Intellectual Wellness

1. I am interested in learning new things. ____
2. I try to keep abreast of current affairs - locally, nationally, and internationally. ____
3. I enjoy creative and stimulating mental activities/games (Sudoku, puzzles, crosswords). ____
4. I am happy with the amount and variety that I read. ____
5. I can analyze, synthesize, and see more than one side of an issue. ____
6. I consider continuing my education beyond college. ____
7. I enjoy and can engage in intellectual discussions. ____
8. I make an effort to improve my verbal and written skill. ____
9. I try to watch television programs that are educational and enriching. ____
10. Before making decisions, I gather facts. ____

Occupational Wellness

1. I manage my time effectively. ____
2. I work effectively with others. ____
3. I am developing the necessary skills to achieve my career goals. ____
4. I have confidence in my job search skills (resume writing, interviewing, etc.). ____
5. I have explored different career options. ____
6. I spend a portion of my time doing volunteer or service work. ____
7. Enjoyment is a consideration I use when choosing a possible career. ____
8. I strive to develop good work habits. (Examples: punctuality, dependability, and initiative). ____
9. I balance work with play and other aspects of my life. ____
10. I take advantage of opportunities to learn new skills which will enhance my future employment possibilities. ____

Now, total your scores in each of the dimensions and compare them to the ideal score. Which areas do you need to work on? How does your score compare with how you rated yourself in the first part of the questionnaire?

	Ideal Score	Your Score
Physical Wellness	40	
Social Wellness	40	
Emotional Wellness	40	
Environmental Wellness	40	
Spiritual Wellness	40	
Financial Wellness	40	
Intellectual Wellness	40	
Occupational Wellness	40	

What Your Score Means

Scores of 35 – 40: Outstanding! Your answers show that you are aware of the importance of this area to your overall wellness. More importantly, you are putting your knowledge to work for you by practicing good habits. As long as you continue to do so, this area should not pose a serious health/ well-being risk. You are likely setting an example for your family and friends to follow. Although you received a very high score on this part of the test, you may want to consider other areas where your scores could be improved.

Scores of 30 – 35: Your health/ well-being practices in this area are good, but there is room for improvement. Look again at the items you answered that scored one or two points. What changes could you make to improve your score? Even a small behavior change can often help you achieve better health and well-being.

Scores of 20 – 30: Your health/ well-being risks are showing. Would you like more information about the risks you are facing and why it is essential for you to change these behaviors? Perhaps you need help in deciding how to make the changes you desire. Help is available from the Office of Health Wellness Promotion, Student Health, CAPS for students, and EAP for faculty/ staff. Through these offices, they will assist you in developing healthier habits that will support and maintain your overall well-being.

What Your Score Means continued...

Score below 20: You may be taking serious and unnecessary risks with your health and well-being. Perhaps you are not aware of the risks you are taking. The resources listed above can help you identify areas of opportunity, develop, and implement life-changing goals.

REFLECTION QUESTIONS:

1. Which dimension(s) of Wellness could you improve?
2. Which dimension(s) of Wellness are you having success in?
3. Which aspects of which dimensions are you ready and willing to work on?
4. What could get in the way of achieving your goal? (e.g., struggling to find time, difficulty feeling motivated)
5. What can help you achieve your goal? (e.g., support of family or friends, seeing results)

Before You Start...

As you consider to engage in counseling, the questions below were created to help you to determine your "Why". What is bringing you to counseling and what are you hoping to get out of this experience.

1. What is bringing you into counseling and coaching?

2. List your issues or problems you want to address?

3. What fears do you have about attending counseling or coaching?

4. What expectations do you have about attending counseling or coaching?

5. Why did you choose to start now?

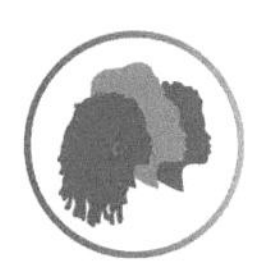

UNDERSTANDING *Counseling vs. Coaching*

Counseling:

- Focuses on both the past and the present.
- Therapy can help heal wounds & trauma from the past.
- Treats a mental health or substance abuse problem (which includes everything from severe issues to minor, short-term issues such as adjustment disorders).
- Because therapy treats mental health or substance abuse problems, it's generally covered by insurance and health savings accounts.
- The client has decreased level of functioning.
- Master's degree required for license & Licensing is required by law Typically generated through illness or dysfunction.
- Diagnostic.
- Healing for maladaptive behaviors and recovery from past traumas Relieving psychological suffering.
- Sometimes covered by insurance Unfortunately stigmatized Practitioner seen as an authority.
- Explores cognition and psychological impact on well-being.

Coaching:

- Focuses on setting & achieving goals in the present and future (doesn't deal with the past).
- Coaching does not involve a mental health diagnosis Coaching helps mentally well people function at a higher level Is NOT covered by insurance or health savings accounts.
- There is no licensing or particular training or credential required to work as a coach Coaches often work online as they aren't limited to working within a state-issued license like a therapist.
- Generally more acceptance of coaching, less stigma Confidentiality not protected by law.
- Orientation on solution and capacity for change Achievement focused/ goal-oriented.
- Certification and credentialing are strongly encouraged Assesses for client's readiness to change.
- Clients are viewed as already whole when entering a coaching relationship Change is self-developed.

PROS & CONS OF Using Insurance

There are multiple reasons for the pros and cons of using insurance to pay for mental health counseling. See them below.

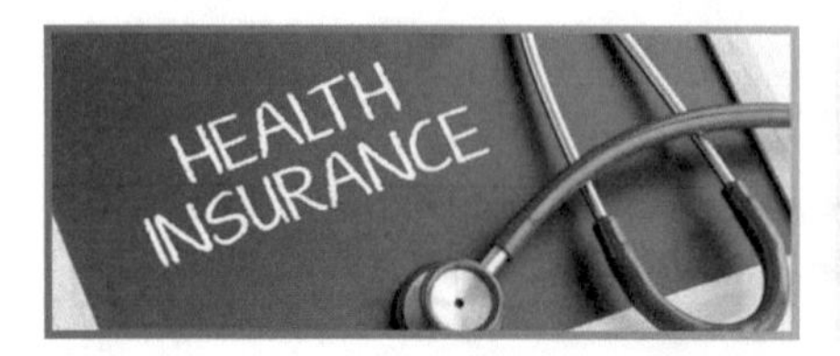

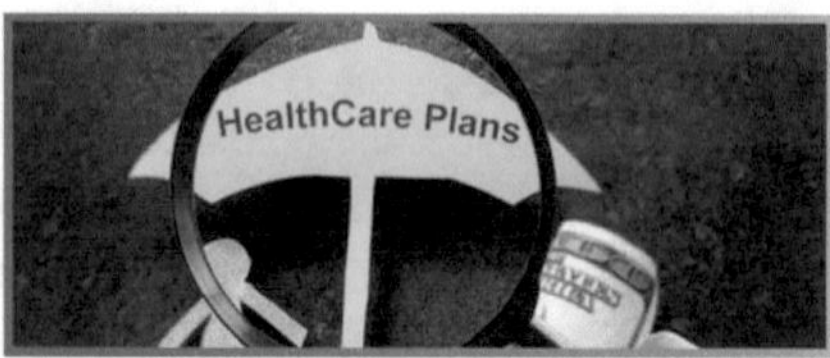

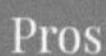

Pros

Cost-Effective

If you have coverage to see the provider you choose, it will probably be cost-effective to use your health insurance to pay for services. With health insurance, you will most likely only pay your co-pay which can range from $10.00 - $50.00. You could possibly pay more if your insurance plan is categorized as a high-deductible plan.

Cost-Effective

Depending on your insurance policy, you may have a $0 to small co-pay only to pay out of pocket and/or deductible.

Cost-Effective

Whether you are self-employed or work for an employer, you effectively pay a lot of money to have health insurance, and it may make sense to get the most out of your benefit package by using insurance for therapy.

Options

A significant portion of therapists does not accept insurance for a variety of reasons. Because of this, having multiple options may be limited in certain areas.

Cons

Required Mental Illness Diagnosis

Insurance companies typically only cover services that are declared as a medical necessity. In other words, your clinician is required to diagnose you with a mental illness in order for the services to qualify for coverage under insurance.

Documented Sessions & Lack of Confidentiality

Any documented health treatment filed through your insurance is required to be recorded on your permanent medical record.

Limited Number of Sessions

Insurance policies often limit the number of sessions you are allowed to attend each year. They may or may not authorize more sessions based on what they determine is a "medical necessity."

Do some insurances have a high deductible that must be met prior to insurance paying for counseling services?

You may have difficulty finding providers that accept your insurance.

YOUR MENTAL HEALTH IS A PRIORITY. YOUR HAPPINESS IS ESSENTIAL.

YOUR SELF-CARE IS A NECCESITY

SELF-CARE ISN'T SELFISH.

FINDING A

Counselor or Coach

Finding the right counselor or coach is SO important, and too often, people just go with the first one available. When you do that, you aren't giving yourself the chance to find someone you truly connect with, and when you meet in real life, you might hate them. I want all of you to have a good experience with therapy, and that's why I put together these tips!

1. Brainstorm what kind of counselor or coach you're looking for. Do you have a preference for gender or race? Do you want someone who has a similar background to you? What about someone who speaks your native language or can incorporate your religious beliefs?

2. Look for counselors & coaches on psychologytoday.com. I like their website because you can filter your search by neighborhood, insurance taken, and by specialty. You can also see where they went to school, their experience, and their areas of focus.

3. After finding a couple of candidates, it's time to cross-reference them with their company/personal website. Check out their bio and see if their approach and goals resonate with you. Sometimes these websites also show what times they practice, office locations, and insurance accepted.

4. When you find a potential candidate, reach out to them by email! You can find their email on psychologytoday.com or on their company/personal website. Introduce yourself, see if they're accepting patients, and ask to set up a free 15-minute phone consultation. I know writing emails can be HARD, so I have created an email template you can use!

5. On psychologytoday.com, you can also see what licenses each counselor or coach has.

IN A COUNSELOR OR COACH

What Am I Looking For?

Making the right connection with a counselor or coach is the most critical factor in the process. We call it therapeutic rapport. In laymen's terms, we call it "a good fit." Just as we have traits and characteristics that we look for in any relationship, some may be important to you as you prepare to enter into counseling or coaching. Use the tools below to identify traits that are important to you.

Take My Insurance	
Availability (Do they offer evening or weekend appts.)	
Personal Attributes (i.e., Race, Gender, Age, Sexuality, etc.)	
Faith & Spirituality (Do you share the same? Do you want it included?)	
What do they specialize in? (i.e., issues & techniques)	
OTHER	

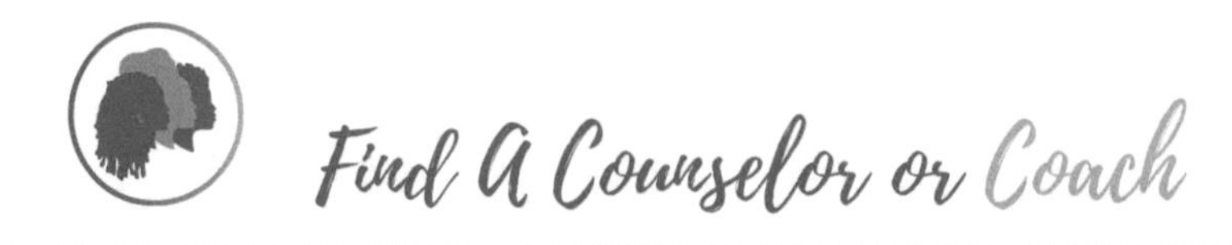

Coaching Directories

- Black Emotional and Mental Health Collective - https://wellness.beam.community
- Noomii - https://www.noomii.com
- Psychology Today - https://www.psychologytoday.com/us/therapists
- Life Coach Spotter - https://www.lifecoachhub.com
- My Coach Match - https://www.mycoachmatch.com
- Life Coach Hub - https://www.lifecoachhub.com
- Bark - https://www.bark.com

Counseling Directories

- Psychology Today - https://www.psychologytoday.com/us/therapists
- Good Therapy - https://www.goodtherapy.org/
- Therapy Tribe - http://www.therapytribe.com/
- Theravive - www.theravive.com
- Christian Counselor - https://www.christiancounselordirectory.com/
- Open Path Collective - https://openpathcollective.org/

  *Reduced Cost Therapy Options for those with financial issues, low or no insurance, and high deductible plans

Counseling Directories for Clients of Color/Minorities

- Therapy for Black Girls - https://therapyforblackgirls.com/
- Therapy for Black Men - https://therapyforblackmen.org/
- Therapy for Latinx - https://latinxtherapy.com/
- Clinicians of Color - https://www.cliniciansofcolor.org/ Inclusive
- Therapists - https://www.inclusivetherapists.com/
- Melanin & Mental Health - https://www.melaninandmentalhealth.com/
- Black Therapist Network - https://blacktherapistnetwork.com/
- My TruCircle - https://mytrucircle.com/
- Caribbean Therapists - https://caribbeantherapists.com/
- Muslim Mental Health - https://therapyformuslims.com/
- Institute for Muslim Mental Health - https://muslimmentalhealth.com/directory/
- Asian Mental Health Collective - https://www.asianmhc.org/apisaa
- Multicultural Therapists - https://findamulticulturaltherapist.com/

International Therapy & Coaching Directories

- The Black Expat - https://www.theblackexpat.com/cm-expert-directory-pro/
- International Therapist Directory - https://internationaltherapistdirectory.com/
- It's Complicated - https://complicated.life/find-a-therapist
- Online Therapy - https://www.onlinetherapy.com/
- The Life Coach Directory - https://www.lifecoach-directory.org.uk/
- The International Association of Professional Life Coaches - https://iaplifecoaches.org/

When Choosing
Your Coach or Counselor...

Trust Your Intuition

Trust Your Intuition

Trust Your Intuition

Trust Your Intuition

Trust Your Intuition

Trust Your Intuition

Trust Your Intuition

Trust Your Intuition

Trust Your Intuition

QUESTIONS TO ASK WHEN INTERVIEWING

A Counselor & Coach

1 Credentials

What licenses and certifications do you have, and which professional organizations do you belong to?

2 Style

How long have you been practicing? Have you worked with clients who had similar issues or diagnosis?

3 Style

What is your general philosophy and approach to helping? Are you more directive or more guiding?

4 Cost

How much do you charge?

Do you accept my insurance?

5

Have you been in counseling or coaching yourself?

Do you receive supervision or consultations?

6 Frequency

How often would you anticipate seeing me? For how long?

7 Feel

What does therapy feel and look like with you?

Can I include my spirituality or religion?

8 Roadblocks

If I feel stuck or things feel unproductive, how will we approach roadblocks?

9 Competency (optional)

Have you worked with a person of color before? What have you done to learn about my specific culture?

10 Conclusion

How will we know when therapy is no longer needed?

Interview Consultation Form

Name of Person/ Practice: ______________________________

Contact Information: ______________________________

RANKING: ____

Name of Person/ Practice: ______________________________

Contact Information: ______________________________

RANKING: ____

Name of Person/ Practice: ______________________________

Contact Information: ______________________________

RANKING: ____

Appointment Tracker

NO.	Date	Time	Format	Link
1.				
2.				
3.				
4.				
5.				
6.				
7.				
8.				
9.				
10.				
11.				
12.				

Appointment Tracker

NO.	Date	Time	Format	Link
1.				
2.				
3.				
4.				
5.				
6.				
7.				
8.				
9.				
10.				
11.				
12.				

Managing Your Medications

For some, medication is or can become a part of your counseling or coaching journey. They can be used to treat a variety of disorders and for both short-term and long-term use. Hence, some people do not require to be on medications for their lifetime while others do. Medications for mental and behavioral health issues can be written by: a) Psychiatrist, b) Physician, c) Psychiatric Nurse Practitioner or Physician Assistant. Some of the aforementioned providers may also provide counseling. It's important to note that not all Physicians outside of mental health are comfortable with writing for these medications.

Below is a chart that you can use to track any medications that may be prescribed to you before or during your counseling or coaching process.

Medication Name (Generic and/or Brand Name) Medication Started?					
What is the medication for? (Purpose and how will it help?)					
How much do I take? (List mg and the quantity.)					
What does the medication look like?					
How often and when do you take your medication? (Any special instructions?)					
Any side effects or issues? (Note symptom(s) & date)					
Notes: (Note changes)					

How to Set Goals

Good counseling or coaching can be life changing. You come to talk and to sort out things in your life. You begin dealing with the recent death of a loved one, decrease bad habits, and don't get stressed out at work. You finally start dealing with behaviors, thoughts, and emotions that have been holding you back.

While counseling or coaching can seem nerve-racking, there are specific things you can do to increase your chances of success. It's possible to take even the smallest or vaguest motivations for therapy and set goals based on them that you can use to track your progress. By following these steps, you can develop a list of personally meaningful goals that can keep your work in therapy focused and productive.

1. Start by identifying broad motives, hopes, and dreams.

At your first session, when they ask, "What brings you to counseling or coaching?" The first thing that comes to mind might be a simple, heartfelt statement like, "I just want to be happy," or "I feel stuck," or "I'm tired of just going through the motions." These statements are too vague to make effective therapeutic goals, but they're a good start. What does being happy look like for you? What specific struggles make you feel stuck? Answering these questions can guide you toward more specific goals. One way to develop goals is to brainstorm and write down as many reasons for coming as you can. Whether you're writing in paragraphs, bullet statements, or making a mind map, the simple process of getting your ideas down on paper (or on a screen) can help you clarify them. It can help to start with a prompt:

- What are some things in your life that you're tired of?
- What are some things in your life that you love and want more of?
- What are some things you haven't done yet that you still want to do?
- Was there a specific problem that brought you to therapy? How and when did it start?

As you build lists and examine your responses to these or other prompts, you may find that certain motives, hopes, or struggles stand out more than others. Explore these more deeply. What you thought your reason was for coming to therapy might not be the most important change you want to make in your life.

2. Choose a theme to focus on.

You might come to counseling or coaching feeling like your life is a total disaster. Where do you even begin? You're having serious problems at work and at home. Your bad habits are affecting your health, your finances, and your relationships. You're having trouble getting on track with anything. It's okay to walk into their office and say, "I'm a total wreck. Can we fix everything?" They will be sympathetic, want to help, and ready to listen to you describe the problems you're having. But you'll be more successful if you work to find specific issues to focus on. If you're falling behind at work and snapping at your partner or children, it might be related to a specific cause that you can address, such as stress or guilt. Counselors are trained to identify root problems and can help you if you're overwhelmed or uncertain how to proceed.

Continued...

3. Narrow your theme into one or more specific goals

Sometimes, it's easy to identify specific goals for counseling or coaching. Sometimes it takes a little more work. Often, it's a matter of finding the right term. "I want to figure out if I'm depressed" is easier to turn into an effective goal than "Something just seems to be wrong." Either one is a fine place to start, but it's easier to identify symptoms of depression than to identify a needle in the emotional haystack of "Something is wrong."

These example goals may give you some ideas:

- "I want to heal from depression and get my hope and energy back."
- "I want to stop having the same fight with my partner over and over again."
- "I want to stop overeating when I'm stressed out and find healthier ways to cope."
- "I want to be creative like I used to be when I was younger. I want to paint, sing, or write again."

Remember that these are just examples and that the range of valid goals is wide and varied. One of the most common reasons people seek counseling or coaching is that they want to be happy but aren't. You can start the process by trusting your instincts and saying what you think the problem might be. You can share suspicions with your counselor or coach that you've been afraid to share with anyone else. When you confess fears like "I think I might be unhappy because I'm in the wrong line of work," or "I'm not sure I want to be with my partner," your relationship with your counselor or coach, and your work with each other will deepen. Even being able to say, "I don't know what I want," can help.

4. Create an action plan to track and achieve your goals.

Once you've identified one or more important goals you want to achieve in therapy, you can work together with your counselor or coach to develop an action plan. Many of them are required to do this as part of the treatment planning process for their agencies. In general, a treatment plan includes major goals, smaller objectives you can use to track your progress toward these goals, and the methods you'll use to facilitate change.

HELPING YOU TO SET
S.M.A.R.T. Goals

Make your goals concrete, measurable, and SMART. The idea of SMART goals comes from corporate management but is a good frame of reference for any process of goal formation. For a goal to be measurable, it has to be specific. Goals that are both measurable and specific are concrete. Time is an important factor in any goal-setting process. Break it up into smaller goals if you're not sure how long it should take to achieve a major therapeutic goal. It's okay if you don't achieve your goals right away; part of the growth process is learning what didn't work and trying again when you don't succeed. SMART goals are:

S	Specific

M	Measurable

A	Achievable

R	Relevant

T	Timely

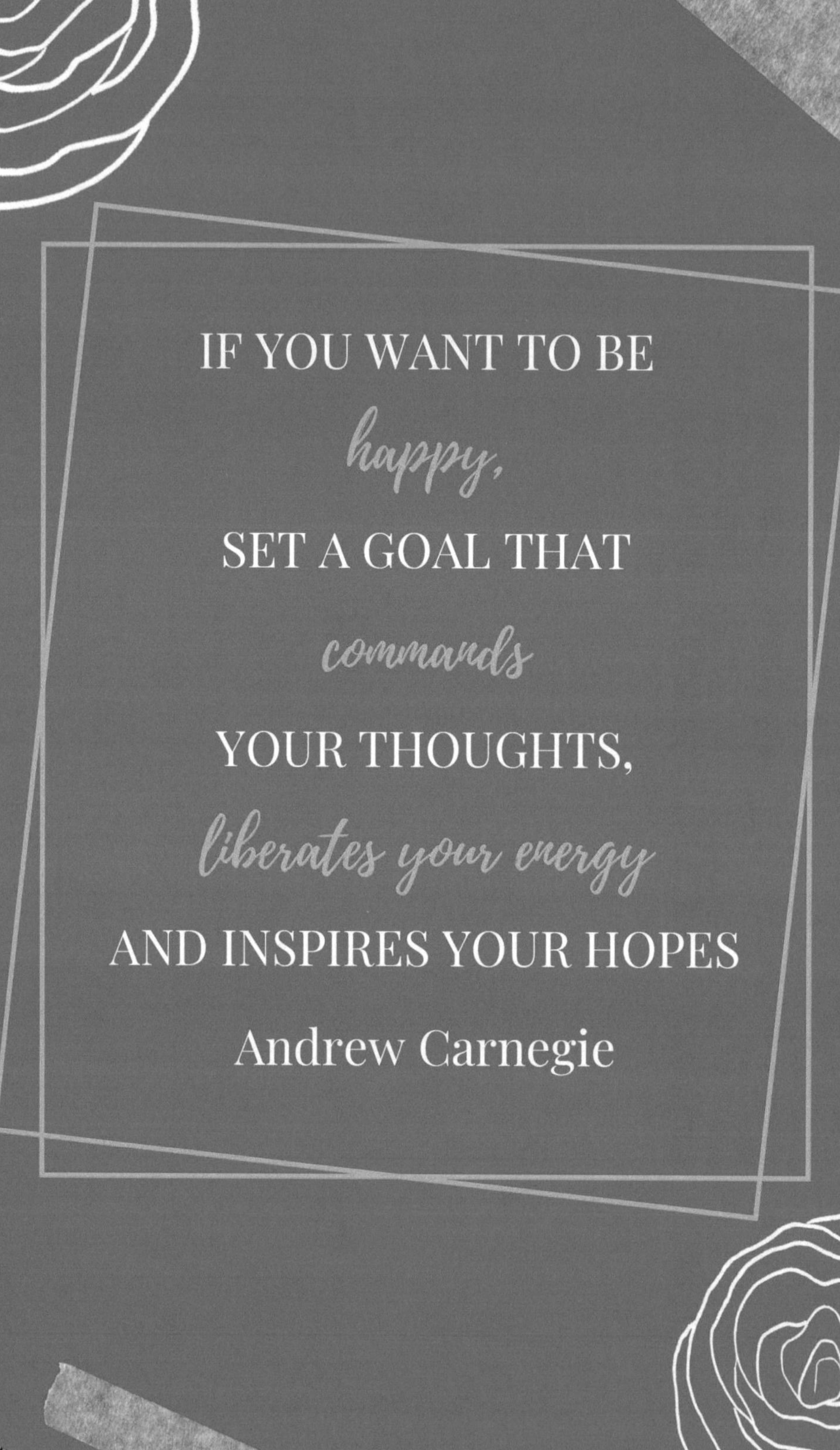
IF YOU WANT TO BE
happy,
SET A GOAL THAT
commands
YOUR THOUGHTS,
liberates your energy
AND INSPIRES YOUR HOPES
Andrew Carnegie

HOW TO GET THE BEST OUT OF

Therapy Tips

- [ ] Be patient with yourself.
- [ ] Think about what you want to get out of counseling or coaching.
- [ ] Go to your first appointment with an open mind.
- [ ] Don't obsess over being polite.
- [ ] Don't keep things to yourself.
- [ ] Be your authentic self.
- [ ] Let your emotions show.
- [ ] Try not to focus solely on symptom relief.
- [ ] Don't worry about the clock.
- [ ] Don't expect your counselor or coach to tell you what to do.
- [ ] Try to schedule your appointments at a good time.
- [ ] Don't expect quick or overnight changes. It's a process.
- [ ] Tell your counselor or coach what's working and what isn't.
- [ ] Be prepared for your sessions.
- [ ] Be committed to attending at least 2-3 sessions when starting sessions with a new therapist.

QUESTIONNAIRE - PART 2

Before You Start...

As you consider engaging in counseling or coaching, the questions below were created to help you determine your "Why." What is bringing you to counseling, and what are you hoping to get out of this experience.

1. How did your problems or issues develop?

____

____

____

2. What things led to the problem or issue?

____

____

____

3. What keeps/ kept the problem going?

____

____

____

4. What thoughts, beliefs, actions, or behaviors prolong it?

____

____

____

5. What behaviors prevented you from being successful in solving the problem or issue?

____

____

____

What to Expect during the Intake Consultation (1st Session)

Completion of paperwork. Paperwork will cover confidentiality, the therapy process, and fees.

Bring in any additional questions that you may have about the process.

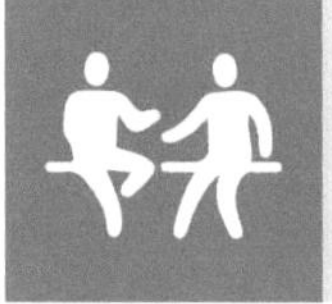

Expect to receive questions asking about your past, who you are & what you want to achieve.

Be authentic & transparent. Don't hide or apologize for your feelings. They can handle it.

Building trust with your counselor or coach is key. If you don't feel like you can trust them, just say so. Ask for a referral for another coach or counselor.

Counseling or Coaching is a commitment. Show up and be engaged each and every time.

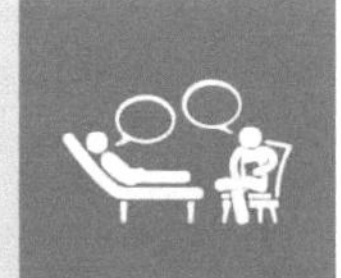

Session Preparation

1. Topics I want to Cover

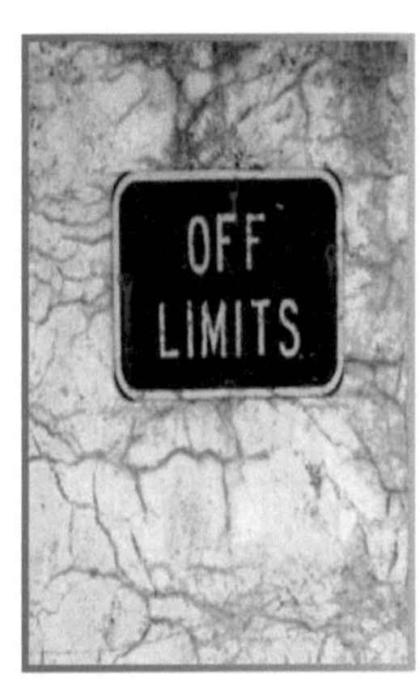

2. Topics I don't want to Cover

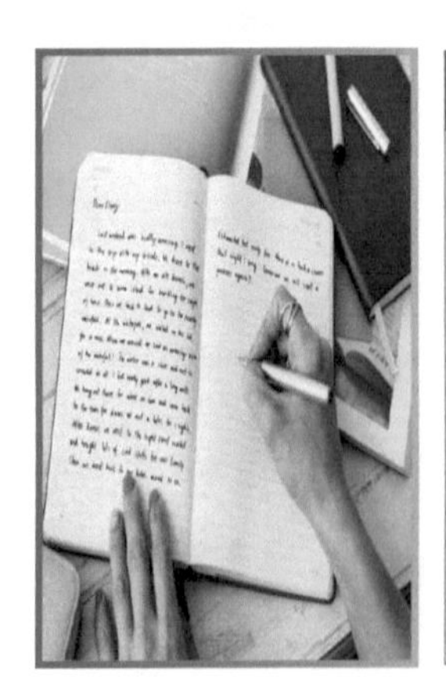

3. Reflections from last session & homework (if applicable)

In - Session Notes

DATE: ____ / ____ / ____

WORKSHEET

Session Reflection

Topics We Covered:	Topics We Did Not Cover:

Likes About My Session:	Dislikes About My Session:

Ah-ha (light bulb) Moments:	Session Reflection:

Homework Assigned:	Topic(s) for Next Session:

SETTING YOUR

Counseling | Coaching Goals

Goal #1	Action Steps
	1.
	2.
	3.
	4.

Goal #2	Action Steps
	1.
	2.
	3.
	4.

Goal #3	Action Steps
	1.
	2.
	3.
	4.

Goal #4	Action Steps
	1.
	2.
	3.
	4.

My Information:

As each counselor or coach is different, you should be able to answer these questions after session #1 or #2.

What is my Diagnosis(es) or presenting problem(s)?	NOTES:
What symptoms are associated with my Diagnosis or presenting problem(s)?	
What are the treatment recommendations for me?	
Is this the right counselor or coach for me?	

Self Check-In

Creating The Narrative. . .

One helpful way to achieve your personal coaching or counseling goals is to evaluate your progress regularly. This form is designed to give you a quick way to track your progress toward your goals and identify any changes you need to make to achieve them.

1. What Have You Accomplished Since Your Last Session? What Were Your Small or Large Successes or New Insights?

2. What are The Biggest Challenges You are Facing Right Now?

3. How are You Addressing The Challenges That You are Facing in Order to Move Forward to Your Goals?

4. How Have I Celebrated Myself Since Our Last Session?

5. What Challenges or Problems are You Facing Right Now & Resources You can Access to Deal With Them?

6. What Would You Like to Focus on In Your Next Coaching or Counseling Session?

Session Preparation

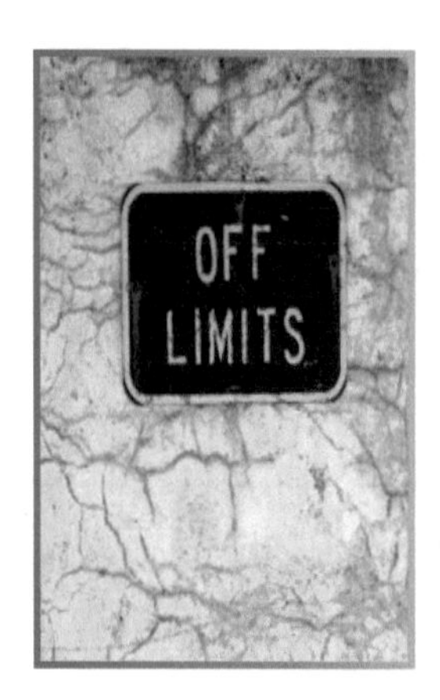

1. Topics I want to Cover

2. Topics I don't want to Cover

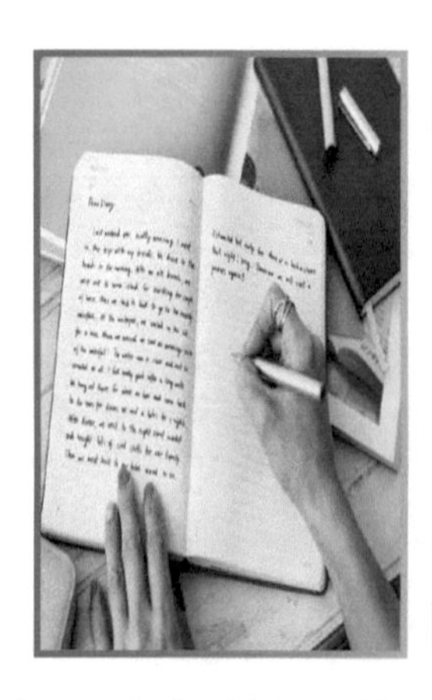

3. Reflections from last session & homework (if applicable)

In - Session Notes

DATE: ____/____/____

- [ ] ____
- [ ] ____
- [ ] ____
- [ ] ____
- [ ] ____
- [ ] ____

WORKSHEET

Session Reflection

Topics We Covered:	Topics We Did Not Cover:

Likes About My Session:	Dislikes About My Session:

Ah-ha (light bulb) Moments:	Session Reflection:

Homework Assigned:	Topic(s) for Next Session:

My Notes

DATE: ____/____/____

Session Preparation

1. Topics I want to Cover

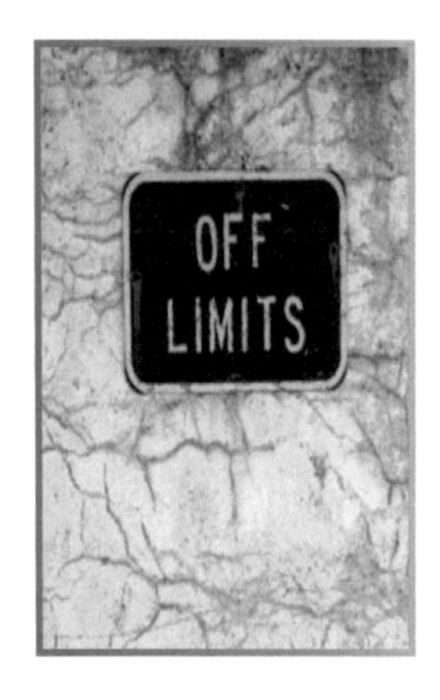

2. Topics I don't want to Cover

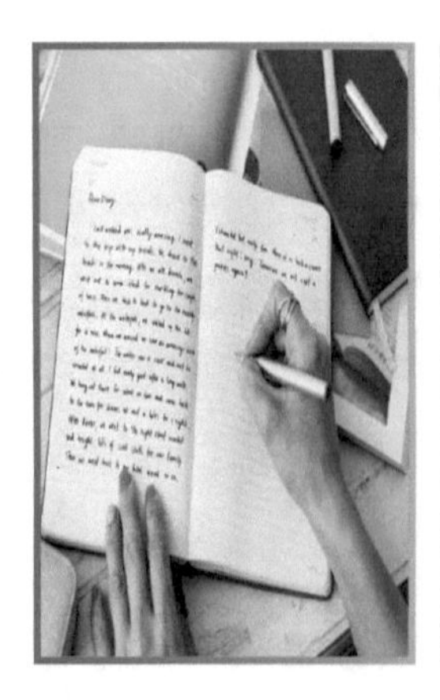

3. Reflections from last session & homework (if applicable)

In - Session Notes

DATE: ___/___/___

- [ ]
- [ ]
- [ ]
- [ ]
- [ ]
- [ ]

WORKSHEET

Session Reflection

Topics We Covered:	Topics We Did Not Cover:

Likes About My Session:	Dislikes About My Session:

Ah-ha (light bulb) Moments:	Session Reflection:

Homework Assigned:	Topic(s) for Next Session:

CLIENT SATISFACTION SURVEY

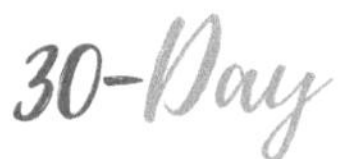

My Opinions About My Changes....

1. My ability to resolve conflicts that arise is:

   Much Improved Slightly Improved About The Same Slightly Worse Much Worse

2. My ability to work towards my goal(s) is:

   Much Improved Slightly Improved About The Same Slightly Worse Much Worse

3. My feeling of respect for myself is:

   Much Improved Slightly Improved About The Same Slightly Worse Much Worse

4. My ability to express loving feelings towards others is:

   Much Improved Slightly Improved About The Same Slightly Worse Much Worse

5. The ability of others (family/friends) to express loving feelings towards me is:

   Much Improved Slightly Improved About The Same Slightly Worse Much Worse

6. My understanding of what is important to me is:

   Much Improved Slightly Improved About The Same Slightly Worse Much Worse

7. My general sense of my future is:

   Much Improved Slightly Improved About The Same Slightly Worse Much Worse

My Experience in Coaching/Counseling:

1. The counselor/coach understood my concerns.

   Much Improved Slightly Improved About The Same Slightly Worse Much Worse

2. My feelings and concerns were validated by the counselor/coach.

   Much Improved Slightly Improved About The Same Slightly Worse Much Worse

3. I was able to raise difficult topics in my counselor/coach sessions.

   Much Improved Slightly Improved About The Same Slightly Worse Much Worse

4. They responded adequately to my questions/concerns about counseling or coaching.

   Much Improved Slightly Improved About The Same Slightly Worse Much Worse

5. I was able to bring up my significant concerns about my life.

   Much Improved Slightly Improved About The Same Slightly Worse Much Worse

6. I am satisfied with my counselor or coach.

   Much Improved Slightly Improved About The Same Slightly Worse Much Worse

Four Change Processes

1. Feelings heal when emotions are conscious and present and we feel safe.

2. Behavior patterns change when we practice new behaviors and stick with them.

3. Ideas change when we become aware that they are erroneous.

4. Unhealthy attitudes are hard to change and require a combination of understanding, persistently talking back to the part of our mind that holds them, and not allowing them to dictate our actions.

Creating The Narrative. . .

One helpful way to achieve your personal coaching or counseling goals is to evaluate your progress regularly. This form is designed to give you a quick way to track your progress toward your goals and identify any changes you need to make to achieve them.

1. What Have You Accomplished Since Your Last Session? What Were Your Small or Large Successes or New Insights?

2. What are The Biggest Challenges You are Facing Right Now?

3. How are You Addressing The Challenges That You are Facing in Order to Move Forward to Your Goals?

4. How Have I Celebrated Myself Since Our Last Session?

5. What Challenges or Problems are You Facing Right Now & Resources You can Access to Deal With Them?

6. What Would You Like to Focus on In Your Next Coaching or Counseling Session?

Session Preparation

1. Topics I want to Cover

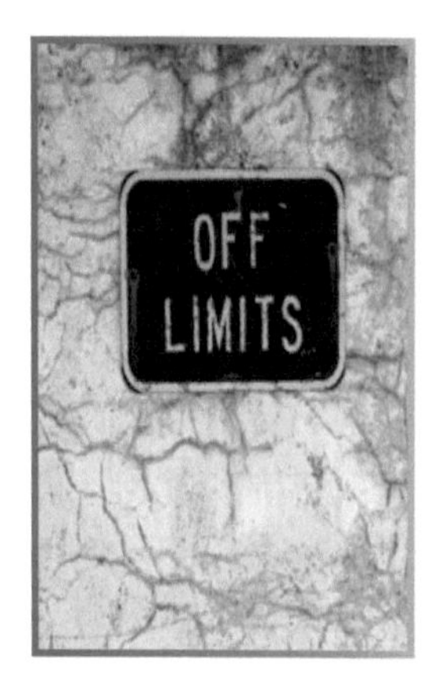

2. Topics I don't want to Cover

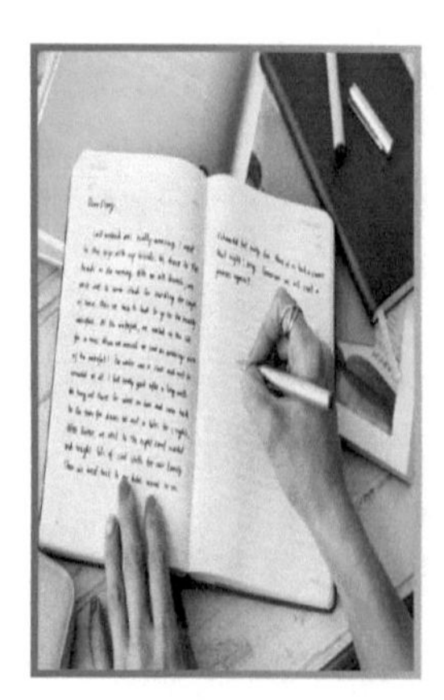

3. Reflections from last session & homework (if applicable)

In - Session Notes

DATE: ____/____/____

- [ ]

- [ ]

- [ ]

- [ ]

- [ ]

- [ ]

WORKSHEET

Session Reflection

Topics We Covered:	Topics We Did Not Cover:

Likes About My Session:	Dislikes About My Session:

Ah-ha (light bulb) Moments:	Session Reflection:

Homework Assigned:	Topic(s) for Next Session:

My Notes

DATE: ___ / ___ / ___

Session Preparation

1. Topics I want to Cover

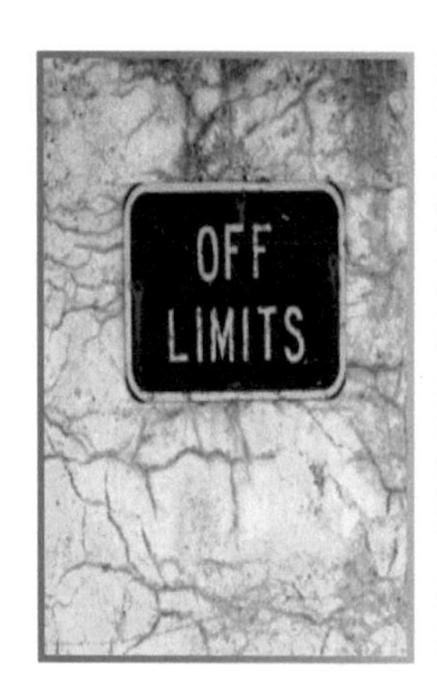

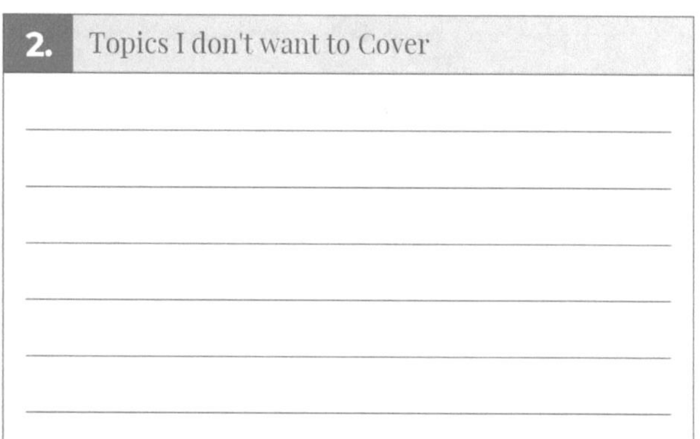

2. Topics I don't want to Cover

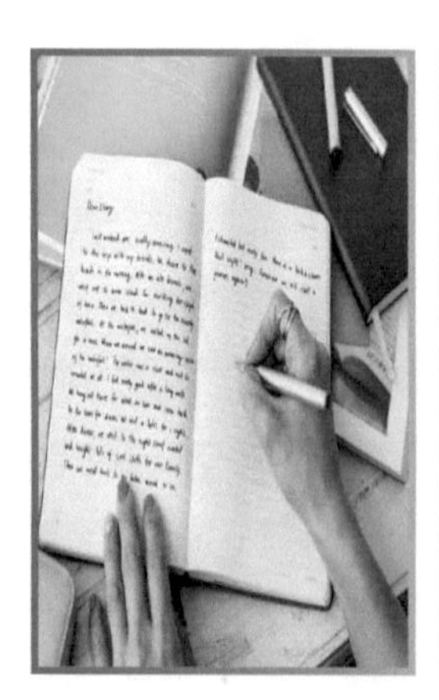

3. Reflections from last session & homework (if applicable)

In - Session Notes

DATE: ____/____/____

- [ ]

- [ ]

- [ ]

- [ ]

- [ ]

- [ ]

WORKSHEET

Session Reflection

Topics We Covered:	Topics We Did Not Cover:

Likes About My Session:	Dislikes About My Session:

Ah-ha (light bulb) Moments:	Session Reflection:

Homework Assigned:	Topic(s) for Next Session:

My Notes

DATE: ____/____/____

Session Preparation

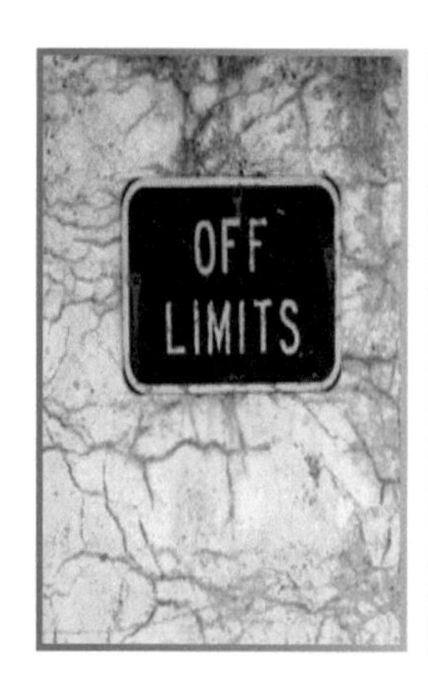

1. Topics I want to Cover

2. Topics I don't want to Cover

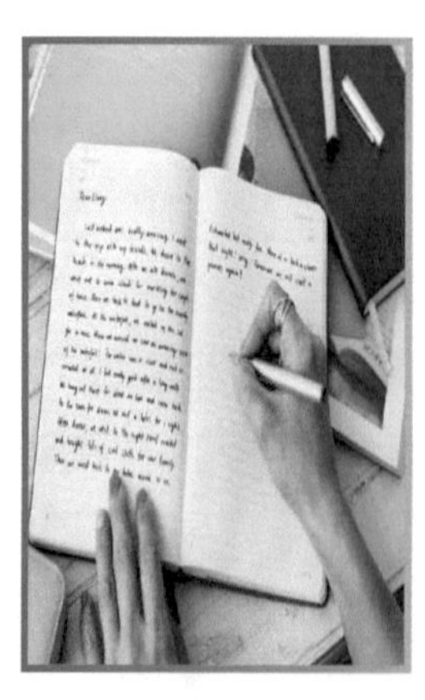

3. Reflections from last session & homework (if applicable)

In - Session Notes

DATE: ___ / ___ / ___

WORKSHEET

Session Reflection

Topics We Covered:	Topics We Did Not Cover:

Likes About My Session:	Dislikes About My Session:

Ah-ha (light bulb) Moments:	Session Reflection:

Homework Assigned:	Topic(s) for Next Session:

My Notes

DATE: ____/____/____

Session Preparation

1. Topics I want to Cover

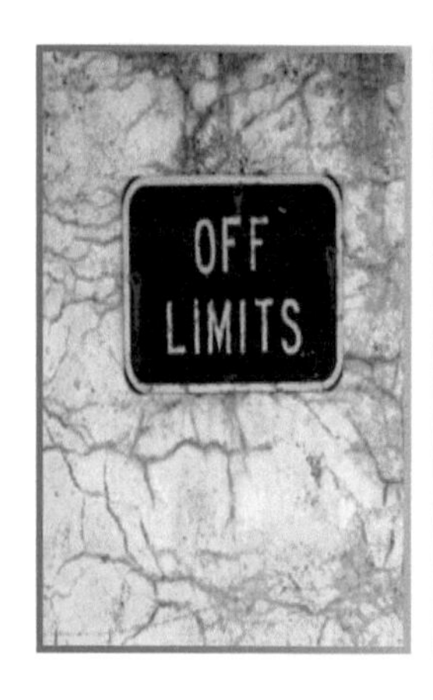

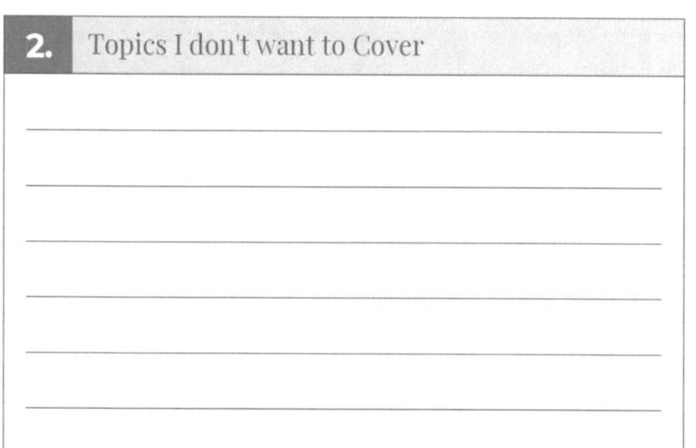

2. Topics I don't want to Cover

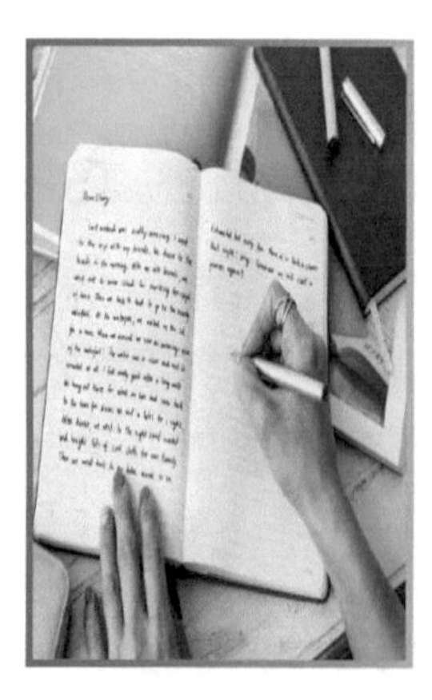

3. Reflections from last session & homework (if applicable)

In - Session Notes

DATE: ___ / ___ / ___

- [ ]
- [ ]
- [ ]
- [ ]
- [ ]
- [ ]

WORKSHEET

Session Reflection

Topics We Covered:	Topics We Did Not Cover:

Likes About My Session:	Dislikes About My Session:

Ah-ha (light bulb) Moments:	Session Reflection:

Homework Assigned:	Topic(s) for Next Session:

My Notes

DATE: ____ / ____ / ____

CHECKUP
60-Day

Use this page to assess where you are 60-days into your counseling or coaching process. Share your responses with your counselor or coach, or use the answers to discuss in your Session Preparation Form.

What Were The Important Sessions of The Month?	Any Changes to Thoughts?

Any Changes to Emotions/ Feelings?	Any Changes to Behavior?

Am I Where I Was/ Began?	Am I Moving at The Right Pace? Do I See Movement?

My Notes

DATE: ____/____/____

Session Preparation

1. Topics I want to Cover

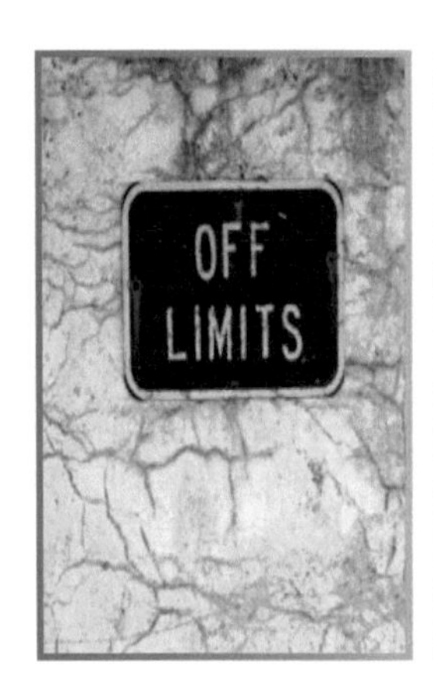

2. Topics I don't want to Cover

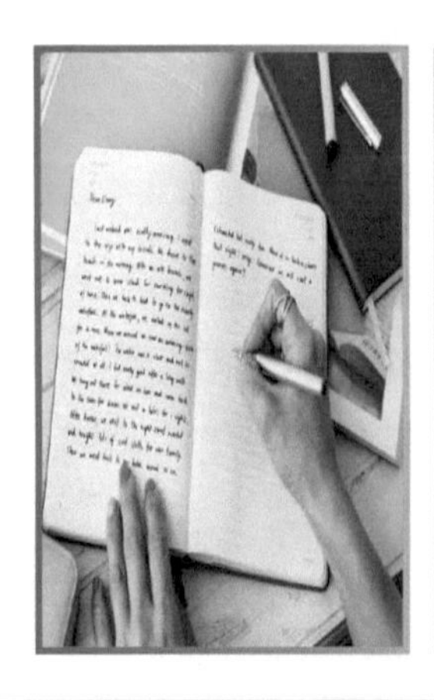

3. Reflections from last session & homework (if applicable)

In - Session Notes

DATE: ___/___/___

- [ ]

- [ ]

- [ ]

- [ ]

- [ ]

- [ ]

WORKSHEET

Session Reflection

Topics We Covered:	Topics We Did Not Cover:

Likes About My Session:	Dislikes About My Session:

Ah-ha (light bulb) Moments:	Session Reflection:

Homework Assigned:	Topic(s) for Next Session:

My Notes

DATE: ____/____/____

PREPARING FOR MY SESSION

Session Preparation

1. Topics I want to Cover

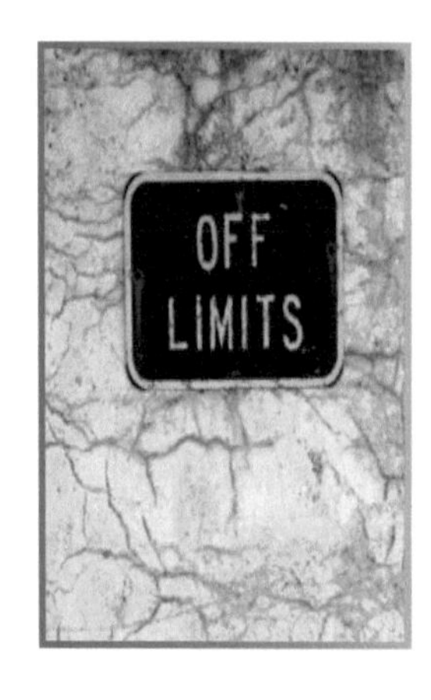

2. Topics I don't want to Cover

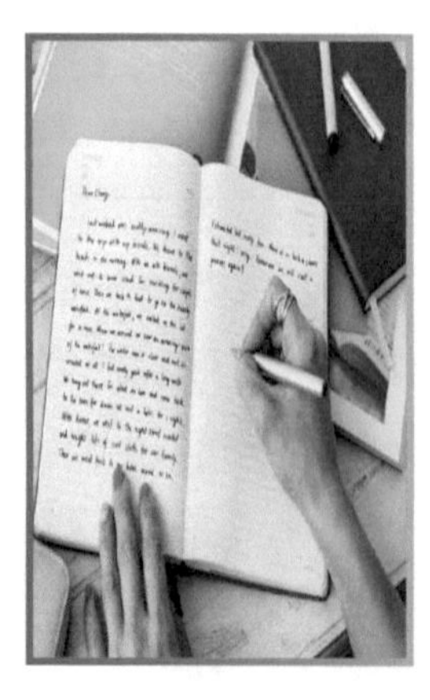

3. Reflections from last session & homework (if applicable)

In - Session Notes

DATE: ___/___/___

- [ ] ______

- [ ] ______

- [ ] ______

- [ ] ______

- [ ] ______

- [ ] ______

WORKSHEET

Session Reflection

Topics We Covered:	Topics We Did Not Cover:

Likes About My Session:	Dislikes About My Session:

Ah-ha (light bulb) Moments:	Session Reflection:

Homework Assigned:	Topic(s) for Next Session:

My Notes

DATE: ____/____/____

CHECKUP
90-Day

Use this page to assess where you are 90-days into your counseling or coaching process. Share your responses with your counselor or coach. Or use the answers to discuss in your Session Preparation Form.

What Were The Important Sessions of The Month?	Any Changes to Thoughts?

Any Changes to Emotions/ Feelings?	Any Changes to Behavior?

Am I Where I Was/ Began?	Am I Moving at The Right Pace? Do I See Movement?

Self Check-In

Creating The Narrative. . .

One helpful way to achieve your personal coaching or counseling goals is to evaluate your progress regularly. This form is designed to give you a quick way to track your progress toward your goals and identify any changes you need to make to achieve them.

1. What Have You Accomplished Since Your Last Session? What Were Your Small or Large Successes or New Insights?

2. What are The Biggest Challenges You are Facing Right Now?

3. How are You Addressing The Challenges That You are Facing in Order to Move Forward to Your Goals?

4. How Have I Celebrated Myself Since Our Last Session?

5. What Challenges or Problems are You Facing Right Now & Resources You can Access to Deal With Them?

6. What Would You Like to Focus on In Your Next Coaching or Counseling Session?

My Notes

DATE: ____/____/____

Session Preparation

1. Topics I want to Cover

____

____

____

____

____

____

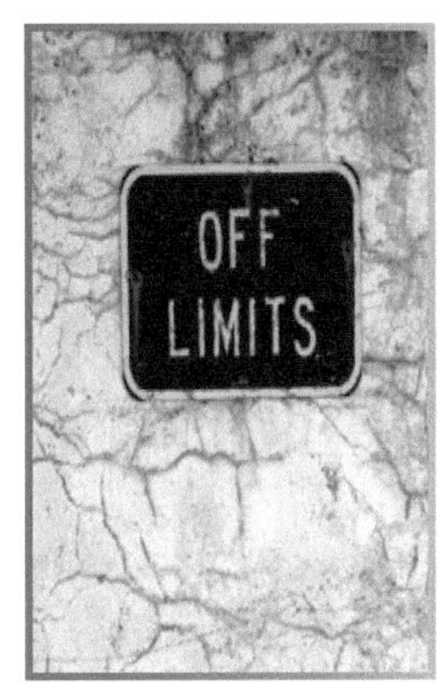

2. Topics I don't want to Cover

____

____

____

____

____

____

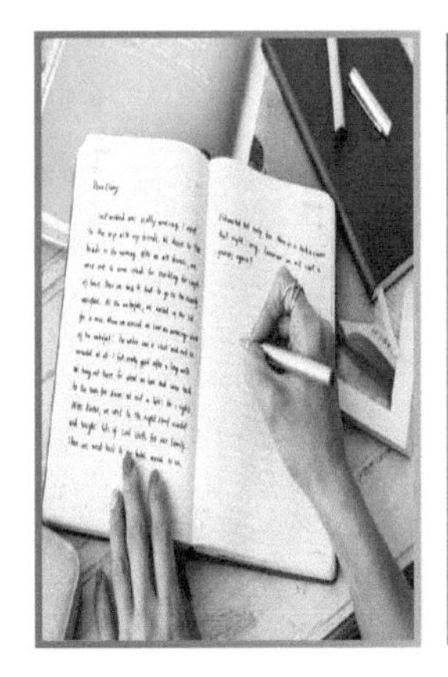

3. Reflections from last session & homework (if applicable)

____

____

____

____

____

____

In - Session Notes

DATE: ___ / ___ / ___

- [ ]
- [ ]
- [ ]
- [ ]
- [ ]
- [ ]

WORKSHEET

Session Reflection

Topics We Covered:	Topics We Did Not Cover:

Likes About My Session:	Dislikes About My Session:

Ah-ha (light bulb) Moments:	Session Reflection:

Homework Assigned:	Topic(s) for Next Session:

My Notes

DATE: ____ / ____ / ____

Session Preparation

1. Topics I want to Cover

2. Topics I don't want to Cover

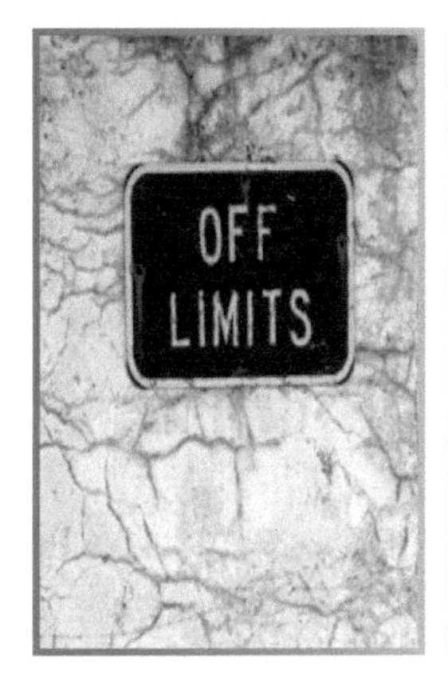

3. Reflections from last session & homework (if applicable)

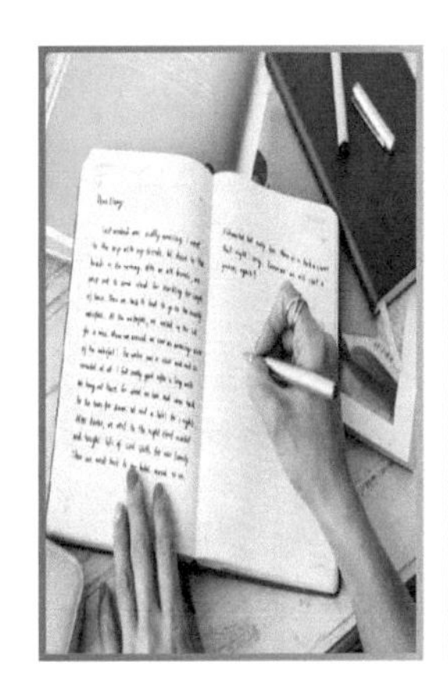

In - Session Notes

DATE: ____/____/____

- [ ]

- [ ]

- [ ]

- [ ]

- [ ]

- [ ]

WORKSHEET

Session Reflection

Topics We Covered:	Topics We Did Not Cover:

Likes About My Session:	Dislikes About My Session:

Ah-ha (light bulb) Moments:	Session Reflection:

Homework Assigned:	Topic(s) for Next Session:

My Notes

DATE: ____/____/____

Session Preparation

1. Topics I want to Cover

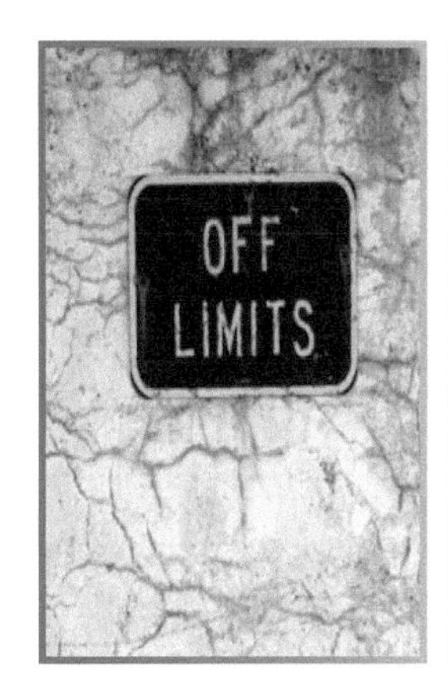

2. Topics I don't want to Cover

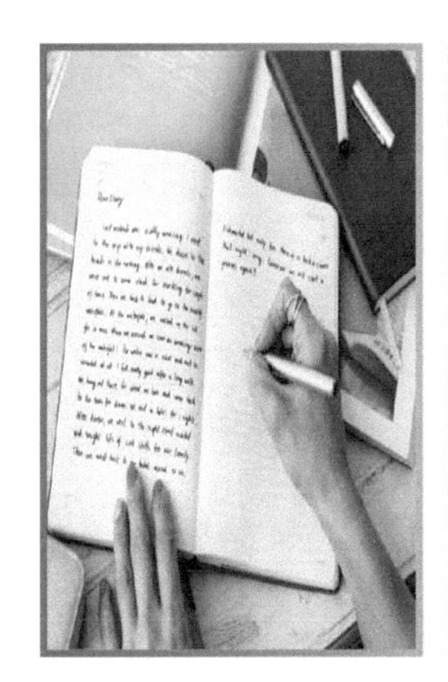

3. Reflections from last session & homework (if applicable)

In - Session Notes

DATE: ___/___/___

- [ ]
- [ ]
- [ ]
- [ ]
- [ ]
- [ ]

WORKSHEET

Session Reflection

Topics We Covered:	Topics We Did Not Cover:

Likes About My Session:	Dislikes About My Session:

Ah-ha (light bulb) Moments:	Session Reflection:

Homework Assigned:	Topic(s) for Next Session:

My Notes

DATE: ___ / ___ / ___

Session Preparation

1. Topics I want to Cover

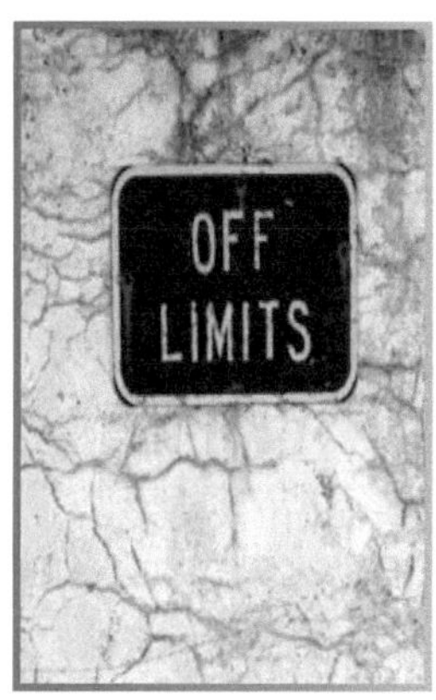

2. Topics I don't want to Cover

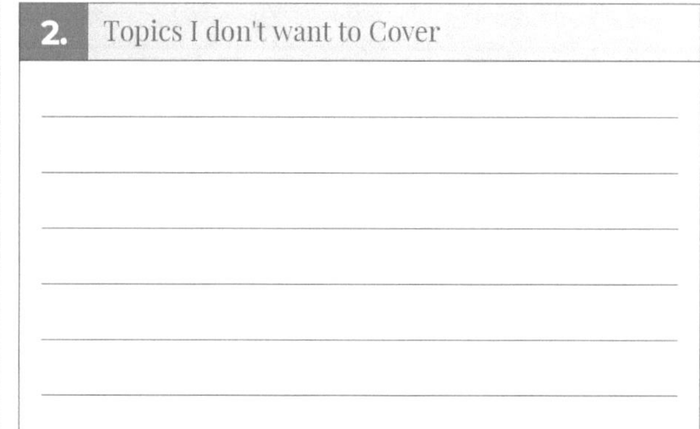

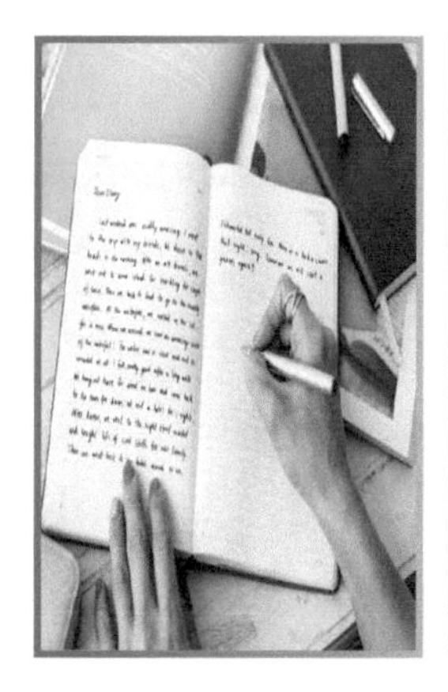

3. Reflections from last session & homework (if applicable)

In - Session Notes

DATE: ____/____/____

- [ ]

- [ ]

- [ ]

- [ ]

- [ ]

- [ ]

WORKSHEET

Session Reflection

Topics We Covered:	Topics We Did Not Cover:

Likes About My Session:	Dislikes About My Session:

Ah-ha (light bulb) Moments:	Session Reflection:

Homework Assigned:	Topic(s) for Next Session:

My Notes

DATE: ____/____/____

Session Preparation

1. Topics I want to Cover

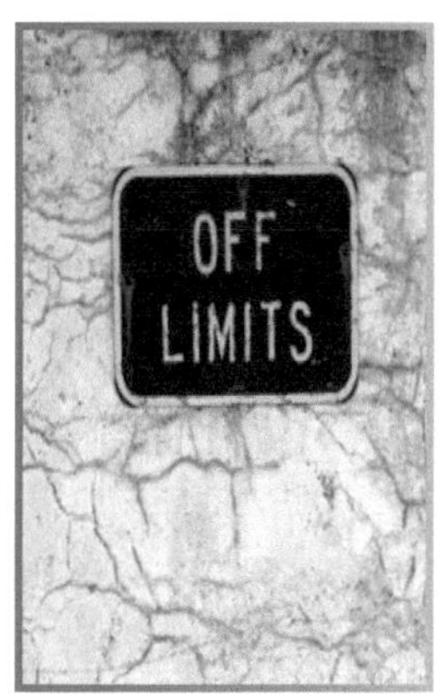

2. Topics I don't want to Cover

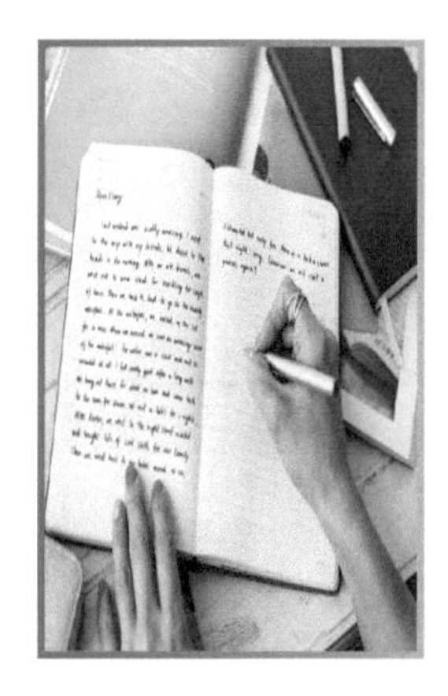

3. Reflections from last session & homework (if applicable)

In - Session Notes

DATE: ___ / ___ / ___

- [ ]
- [ ]
- [ ]
- [ ]
- [ ]
- [ ]

WORKSHEET

Session Reflection

Topics We Covered:	Topics We Did Not Cover:

Likes About My Session:	Dislikes About My Session:

Ah-ha (light bulb) Moments:	Session Reflection:

Homework Assigned:	Topic(s) for Next Session:

My Notes

DATE: ____/____/____

Session Preparation

1. Topics I want to Cover

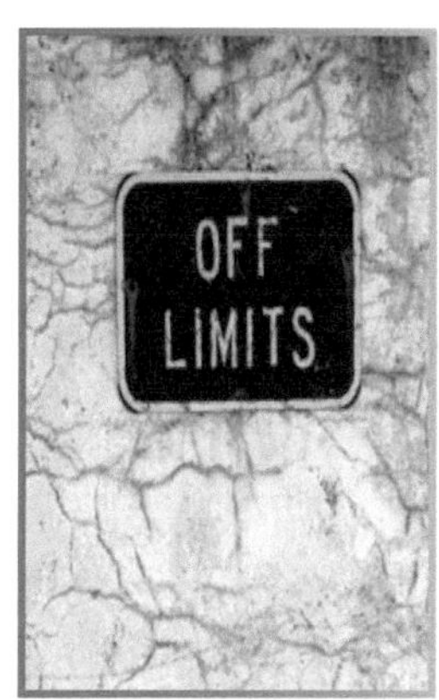

2. Topics I don't want to Cover

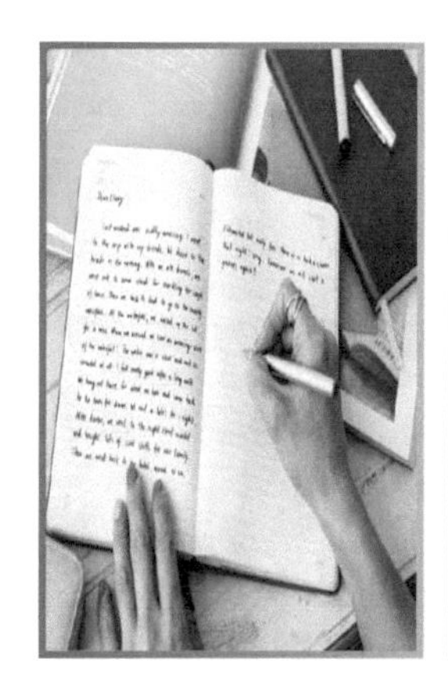

3. Reflections from last session & homework (if applicable)

In - Session Notes

DATE: ___/___/___

- [ ] ______

- [ ] ______

- [ ] ______

- [ ] ______

- [ ] ______

- [ ] ______

WORKSHEET

Session Reflection

Topics We Covered:	Topics We Did Not Cover:

Likes About My Session:	Dislikes About My Session:

Ah-ha (light bulb) Moments:	Session Reflection:

Homework Assigned:	Topic(s) for Next Session:

My Notes

DATE: ____/____/____

Session Preparation

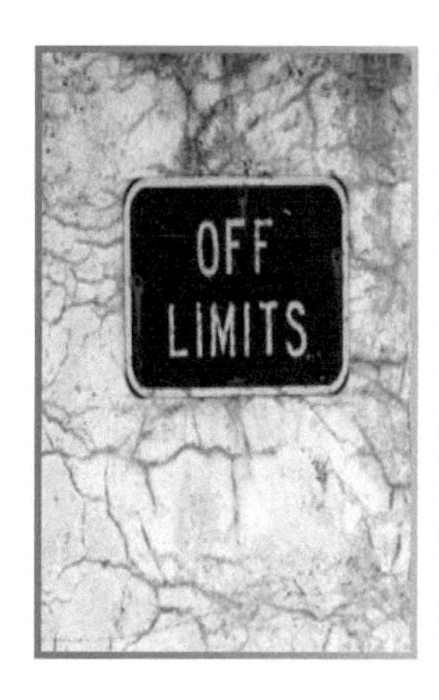

1. Topics I want to Cover

2. Topics I don't want to Cover

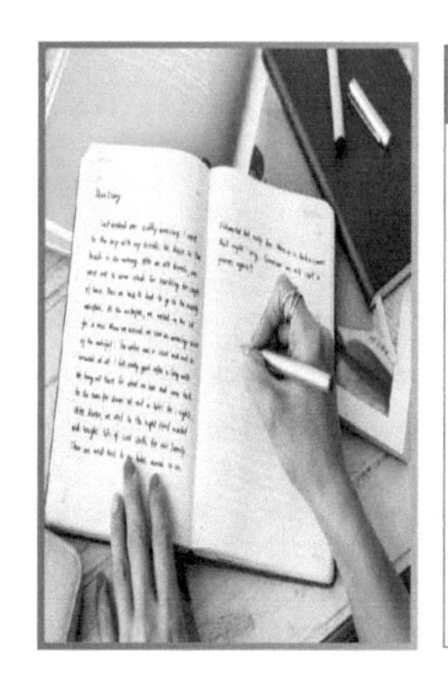

3. Reflections from last session & homework (if applicable)

In - Session Notes

DATE: ____/____/____

- [ ]

- [ ]

- [ ]

- [ ]

- [ ]

- [ ]

WORKSHEET

Session Reflection

Topics We Covered:	Topics We Did Not Cover:

Likes About My Session:	Dislikes About My Session:

Ah-ha (light bulb) Moments:	Session Reflection:

Homework Assigned:	Topic(s) for Next Session:

My Notes

DATE: ___ / ___ / ___

Session Preparation

1. Topics I want to Cover

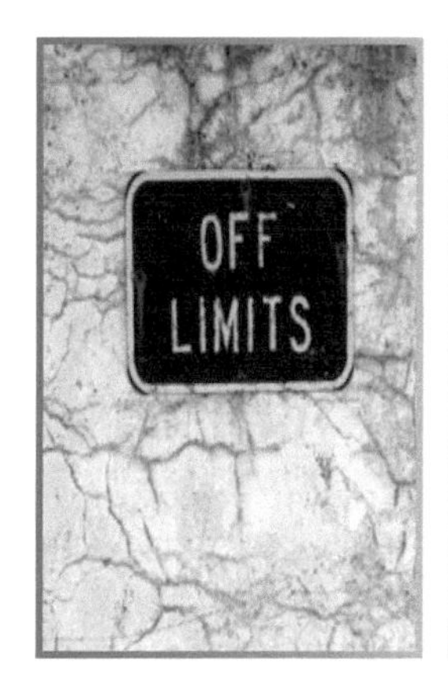

2. Topics I don't want to Cover

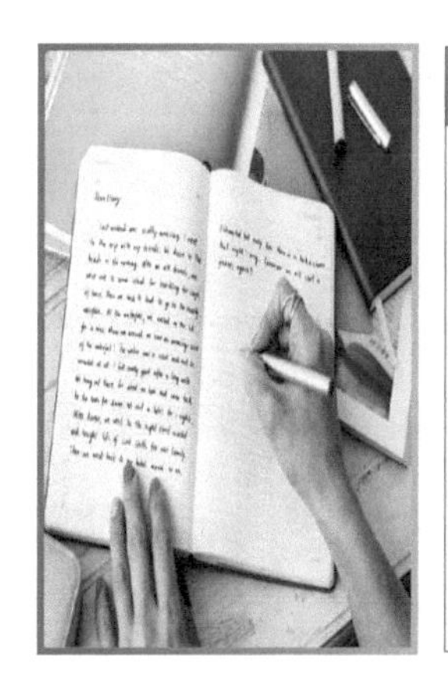

3. Reflections from last session & homework (if applicable)

In - Session Notes

DATE: ____/____/____

- [ ]

- [ ]

- [ ]

- [ ]

- [ ]

- [ ]

WORKSHEET

Session Reflection

Topics We Covered:	Topics We Did Not Cover:

Likes About My Session:	Dislikes About My Session:

Ah-ha (light bulb) Moments:	Session Reflection:

Homework Assigned:	Topic(s) for Next Session:

My Notes

DATE: ____/____/____

Session Preparation

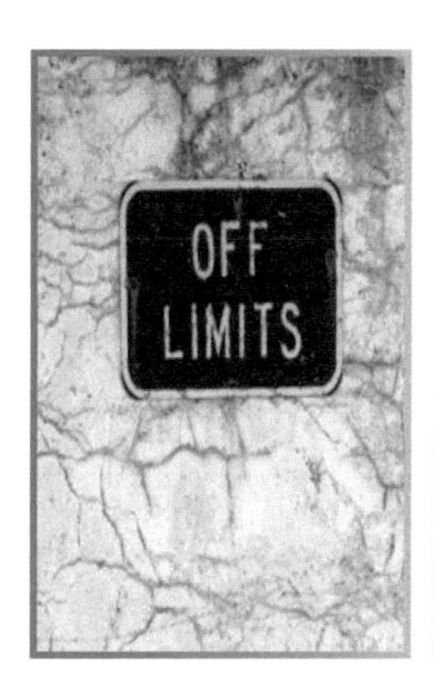

1. Topics I want to Cover

2. Topics I don't want to Cover

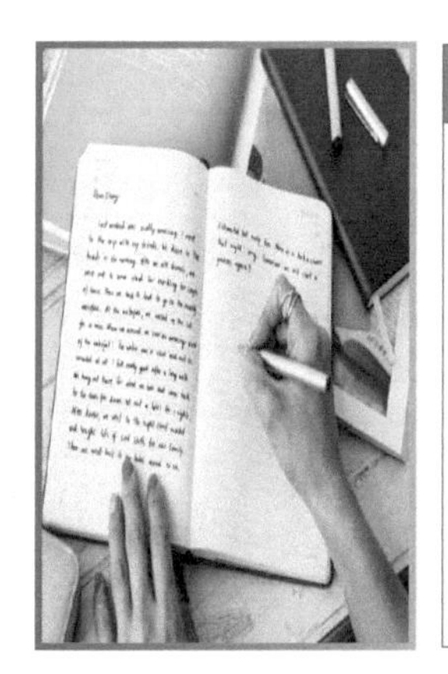

3. Reflections from last session & homework (if applicable)

In - Session Notes

DATE: ____/____/____

- [ ]
- [ ]
- [ ]
- [ ]
- [ ]
- [ ]

WORKSHEET

Session Reflection

Topics We Covered:	Topics We Did Not Cover:

Likes About My Session:	Dislikes About My Session:

Ah-ha (light bulb) Moments:	Session Reflection:

Homework Assigned:	Topic(s) for Next Session:

My Notes

DATE: ____ / ____ / ____

Session Preparation

1. Topics I want to Cover

2. Topics I don't want to Cover

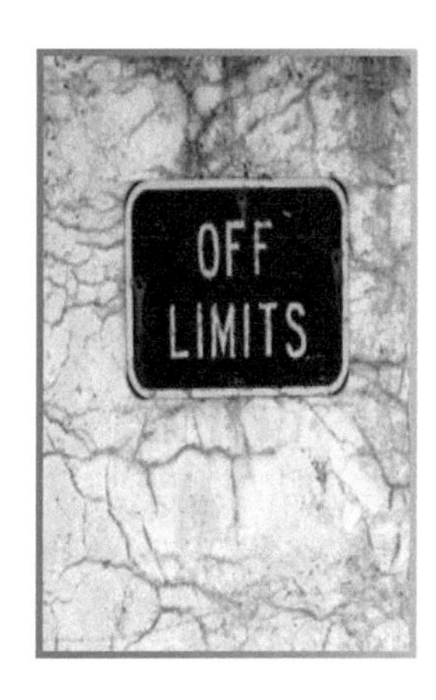

3. Reflections from last session & homework (if applicable)

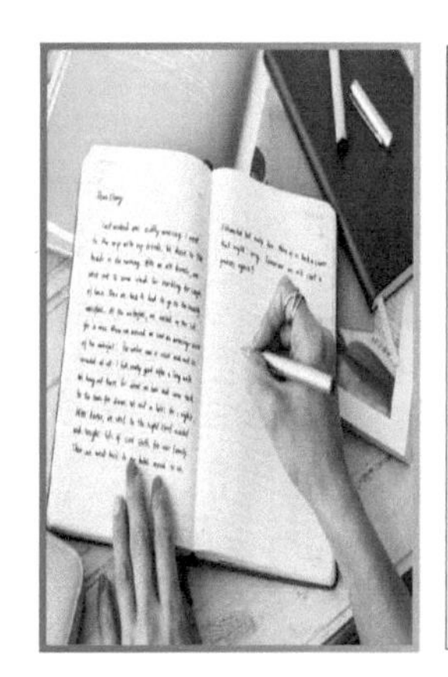

In - Session Notes

DATE: ____/____/____

- [ ] ____
- [ ] ____
- [ ] ____
- [ ] ____
- [ ] ____
- [ ] ____

WORKSHEET

Session Reflection

Topics We Covered:	Topics We Did Not Cover:

Likes About My Session:	Dislikes About My Session:

Ah-ha (light bulb) Moments:	Session Reflection:

Homework Assigned:	Topic(s) for Next Session:

My Notes

DATE: ____/____/____

CHECKUP
6-Month

Use this page to assess where you are 6 months into your counseling or coaching process. Share your responses with your counselor or coach, or use the answers to discuss in your Session Preparation Form.

What Were The Important Sessions of The Month?	Any Changes to Thoughts?

Any Changes to Emotions/ Feelings?	Any Changes to Behavior?

Am I Where I Was/ Began?	Am I Moving at The Right Pace? Do I See Movement?

My Notes

DATE: ____/____/____

Session Preparation

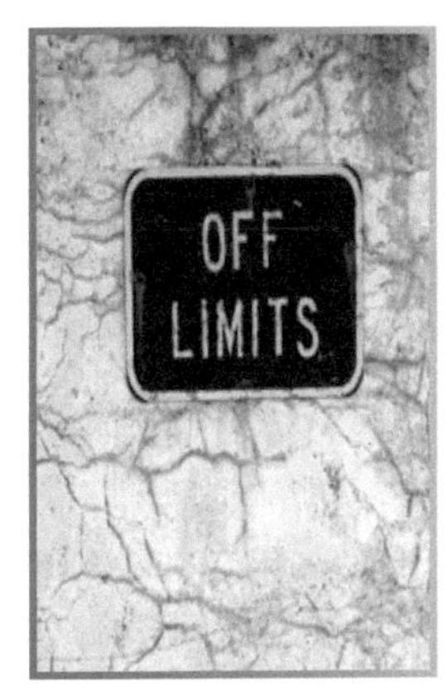

1. Topics I want to Cover

2. Topics I don't want to Cover

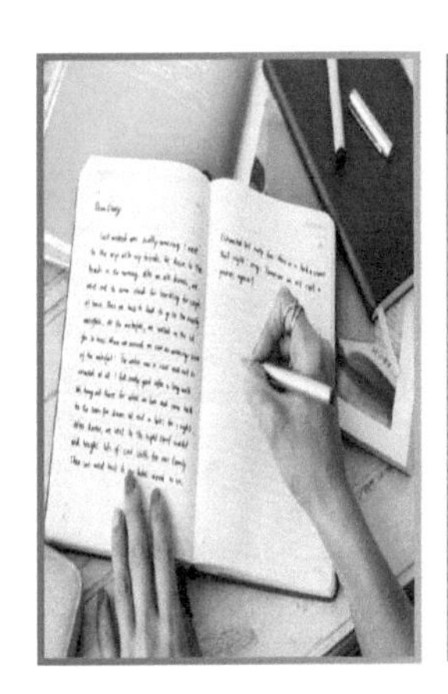

3. Reflections from last session & homework (if applicable)

In - Session Notes

DATE: ____ / ____ / ____

WORKSHEET

Session Reflection

Topics We Covered:	Topics We Did Not Cover:

Likes About My Session:	Dislikes About My Session:

Ah-ha (light bulb) Moments:	Session Reflection:

Homework Assigned:	Topic(s) for Next Session:

My Notes

DATE: ____/____/____

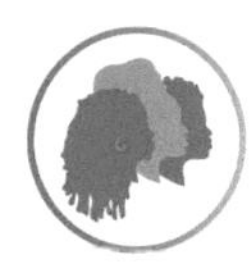

Session Preparation

1. Topics I want to Cover

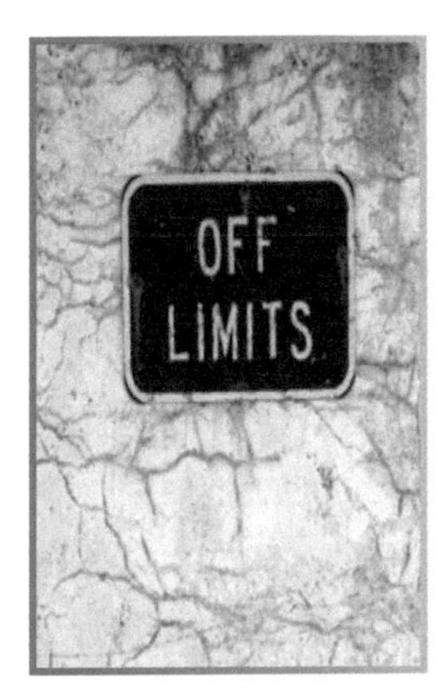

2. Topics I don't want to Cover

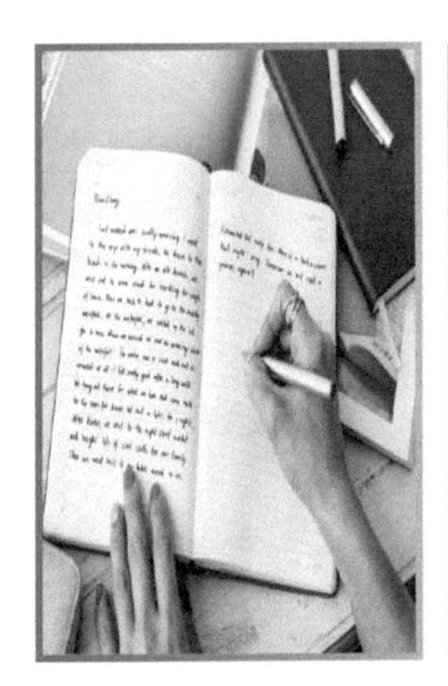

3. Reflections from last session & homework (if applicable)

In - Session Notes

DATE: ____/____/____

☐ ______

☐ ______

☐ ______

☐ ______

☐ ______

☐ ______

WORKSHEET

Session Reflection

Topics We Covered:	Topics We Did Not Cover:

Likes About My Session:	Dislikes About My Session:

Ah-ha (light bulb) Moments:	Session Reflection:

Homework Assigned:	Topic(s) for Next Session:

My Notes

DATE: ___ / ___ / ___

Session Preparation

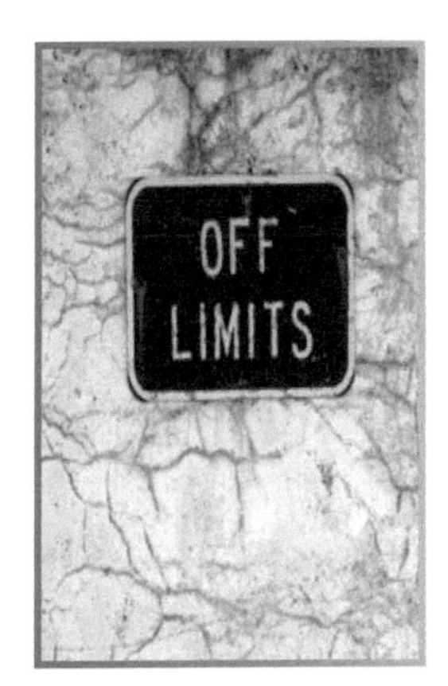

1. Topics I want to Cover

2. Topics I don't want to Cover

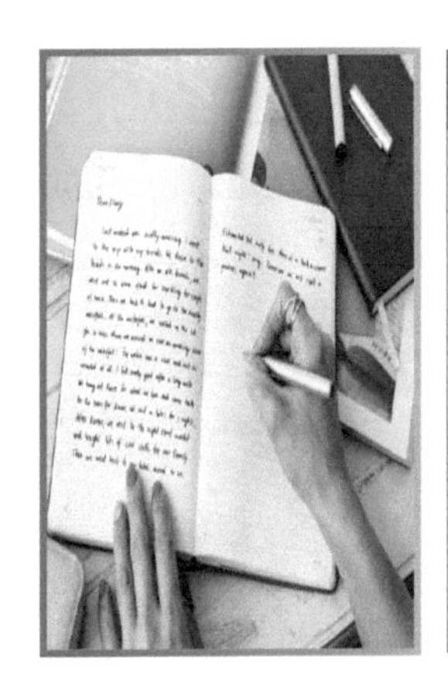

3. Reflections from last session & homework (if applicable)

In - Session Notes

DATE: ____/____/____

- [ ] ____
- [ ] ____
- [ ] ____
- [ ] ____
- [ ] ____
- [ ] ____

WORKSHEET

Session Reflection

Topics We Covered:	Topics We Did Not Cover:

Likes About My Session:	Dislikes About My Session:

Ah-ha (light bulb) Moments:	Session Reflection:

Homework Assigned:	Topic(s) for Next Session:

My Notes

DATE: ____/____/____

Session Preparation

1. Topics I want to Cover

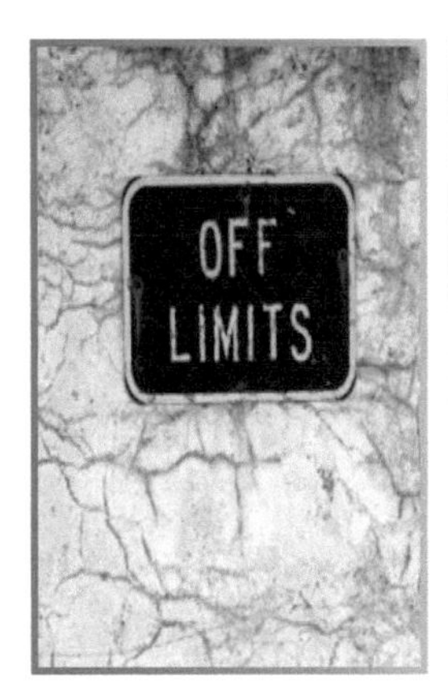

2. Topics I don't want to Cover

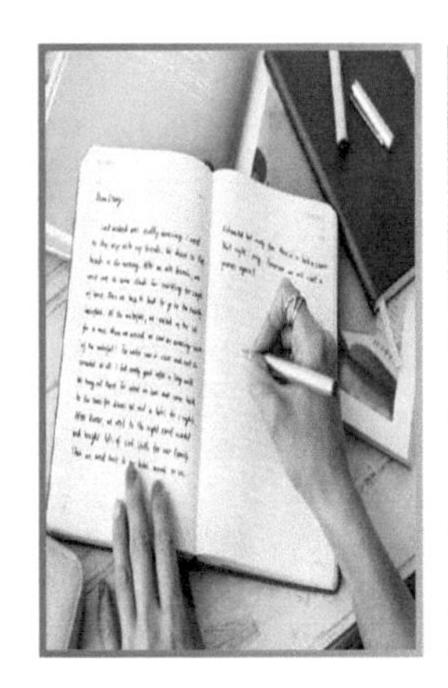

3. Reflections from last session & homework (if applicable)

In - Session Notes

DATE: ____/____/____

- [ ] ______________________________
- [ ] ______________________________
- [ ] ______________________________
- [ ] ______________________________
- [ ] ______________________________
- [ ] ______________________________

WORKSHEET

Session Reflection

Topics We Covered:	Topics We Did Not Cover:

Likes About My Session:	Dislikes About My Session:

Ah-ha (light bulb) Moments:	Session Reflection:

Homework Assigned:	Topic(s) for Next Session:

My Notes

DATE: ____/____/____

Session Preparation

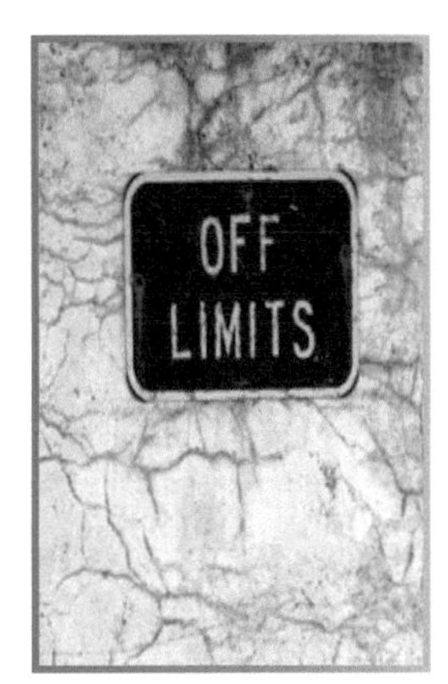

1. Topics I want to Cover

2. Topics I don't want to Cover

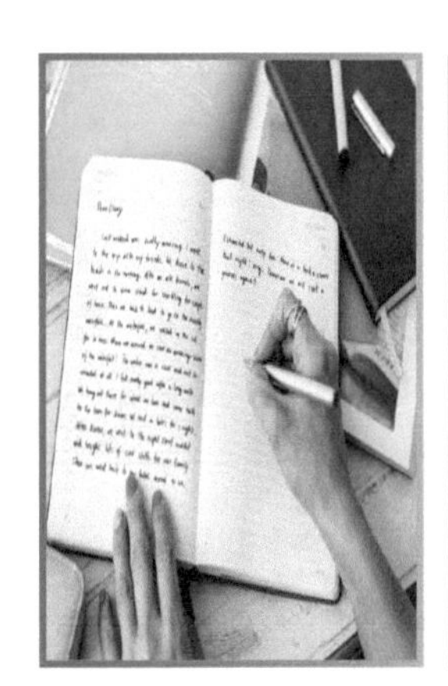

3. Reflections from last session & homework (if applicable)

In - Session Notes

DATE: ___/___/___

- [ ]

- [ ]

- [ ]

- [ ]

- [ ]

- [ ]

WORKSHEET

Session Reflection

Topics We Covered:	Topics We Did Not Cover:

Likes About My Session:	Dislikes About My Session:

Ah-ha (light bulb) Moments:	Session Reflection:

Homework Assigned:	Topic(s) for Next Session:

My Notes

DATE: ____/____/____

Session Preparation

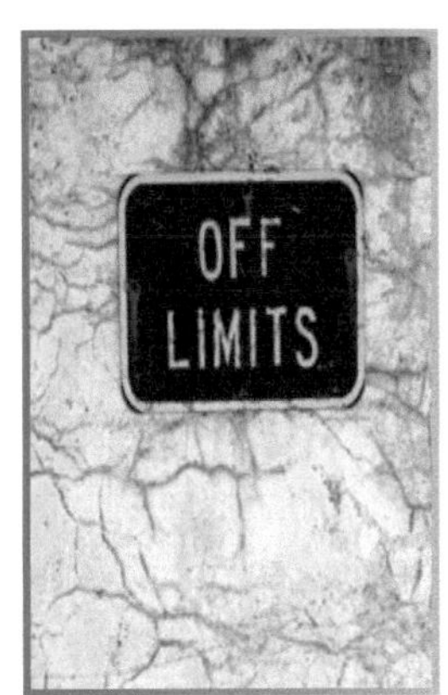

1. Topics I want to Cover

2. Topics I don't want to Cover

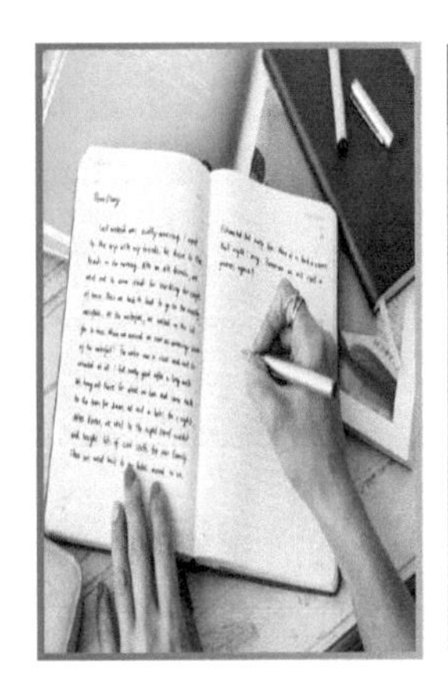

3. Reflections from last session & homework (if applicable)

In - Session Notes

DATE: ___ / ___ / ___

- [ ]
- [ ]
- [ ]
- [ ]
- [ ]
- [ ]

WORKSHEET

Session Reflection

Topics We Covered:	Topics We Did Not Cover:

Likes About My Session:	Dislikes About My Session:

Ah-ha (light bulb) Moments:	Session Reflection:

Homework Assigned:	Topic(s) for Next Session:

My Notes

DATE: ____/____/____

Session Preparation

1. Topics I want to Cover

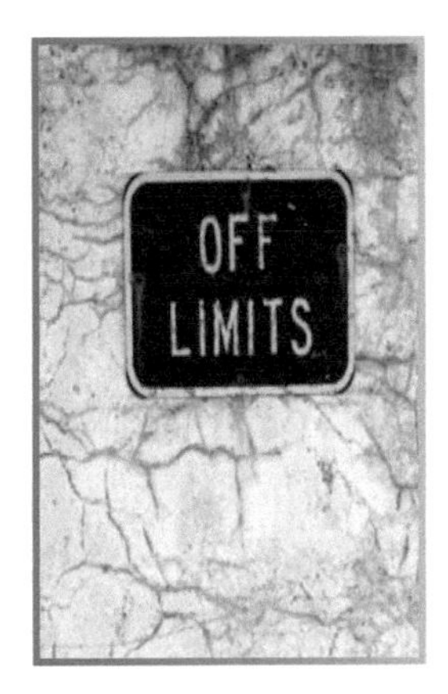

2. Topics I don't want to Cover

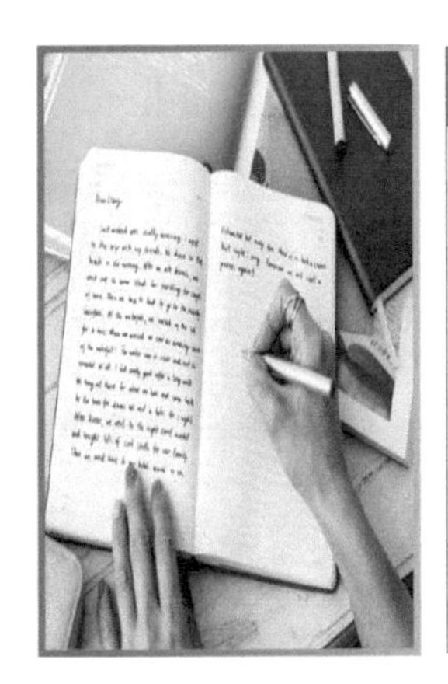

3. Reflections from last session & homework (if applicable)

In - Session Notes

DATE: ____/____/____

- [ ] ______
- [ ] ______
- [ ] ______
- [ ] ______
- [ ] ______
- [ ] ______

WORKSHEET

Session Reflection

Topics We Covered:	Topics We Did Not Cover:

Likes About My Session:	Dislikes About My Session:

Ah-ha (light bulb) Moments:	Session Reflection:

Homework Assigned:	Topic(s) for Next Session:

My Notes

DATE: ____ / ____ / ____

Session Preparation

1. Topics I want to Cover

2. Topics I don't want to Cover

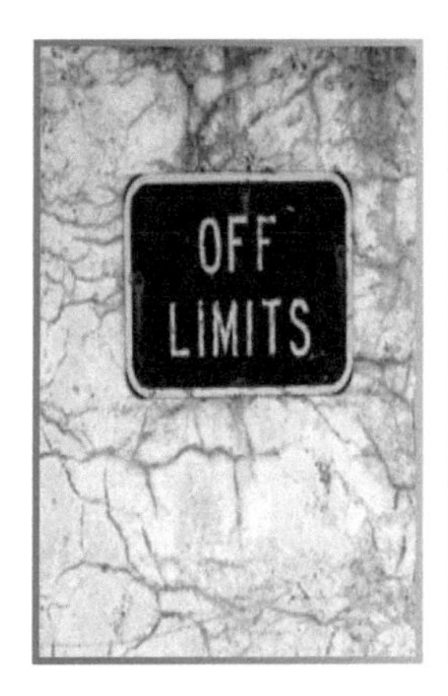

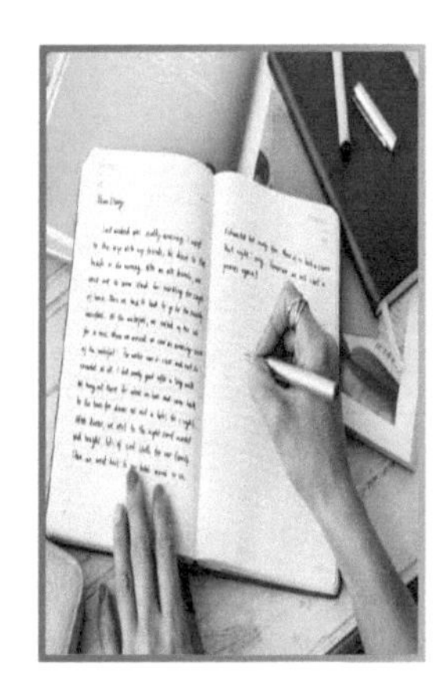

3. Reflections from last session & homework (if applicable)

In - Session Notes

DATE: ____ / ____ / ____

- [ ]

- [ ]

- [ ]

- [ ]

- [ ]

- [ ]

WORKSHEET

Session Reflection

Topics We Covered:	Topics We Did Not Cover:

Likes About My Session:	Dislikes About My Session:

Ah-ha (light bulb) Moments:	Session Reflection:

Homework Assigned:	Topic(s) for Next Session:

My Notes

DATE: ____/____/____

Session Preparation

1. Topics I want to Cover

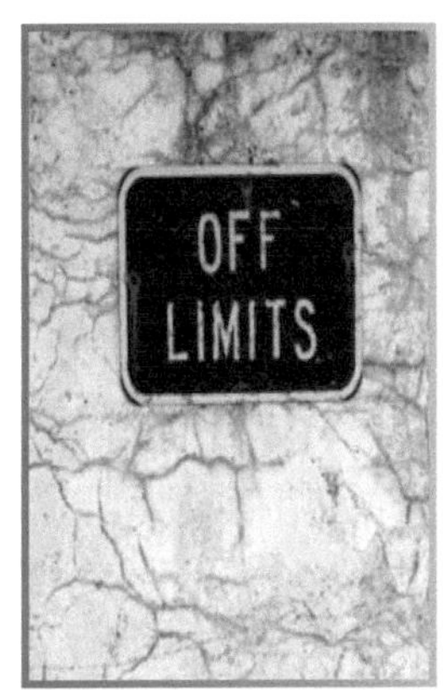

2. Topics I don't want to Cover

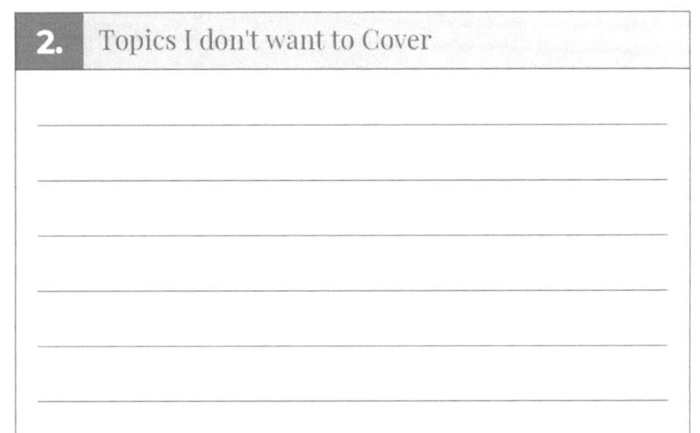

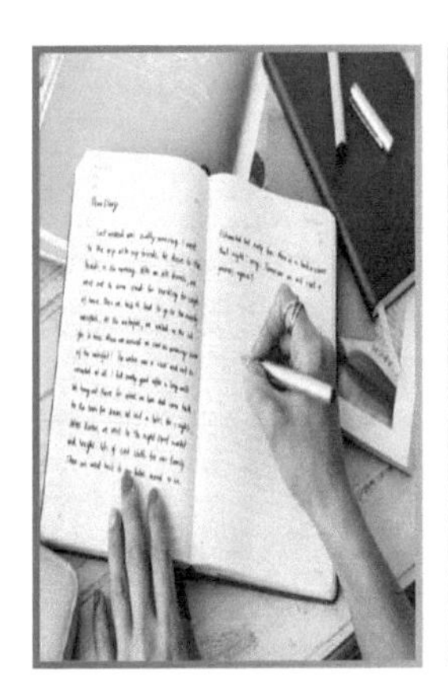

3. Reflections from last session & homework (if applicable)

In - Session Notes

DATE: ___/___/___

- [ ]

- [ ]

- [ ]

- [ ]

- [ ]

- [ ]

WORKSHEET

Session Reflection

Topics We Covered:	Topics We Did Not Cover:

Likes About My Session:	Dislikes About My Session:

Ah-ha (light bulb) Moments:	Session Reflection:

Homework Assigned:	Topic(s) for Next Session:

My Notes

DATE: ____/____/____

Session Preparation

1. Topics I want to Cover

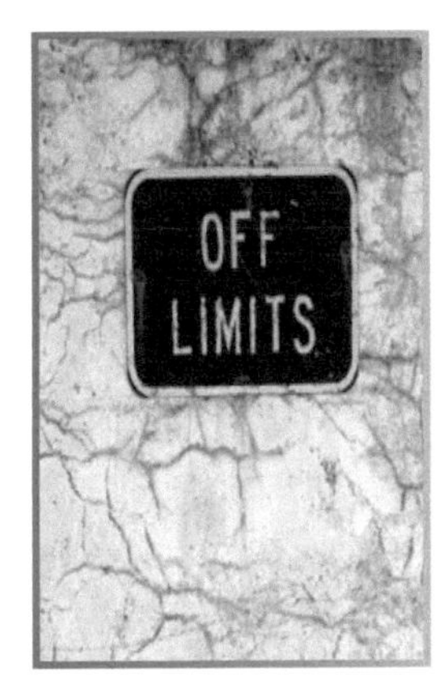

2. Topics I don't want to Cover

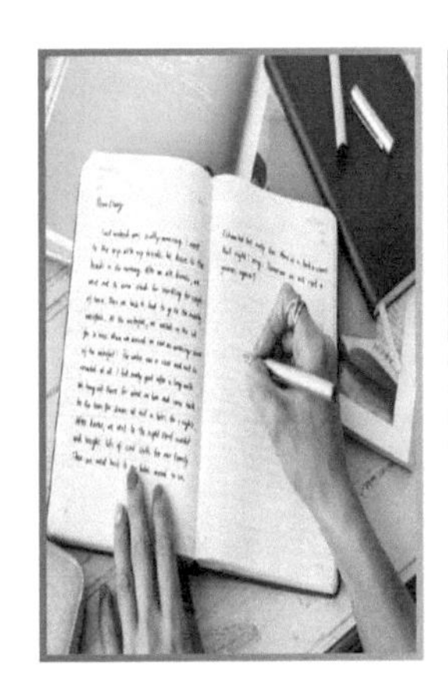

3. Reflections from last session & homework (if applicable)

In - Session Notes

DATE: ___ / ___ / ___

- [ ]
- [ ]
- [ ]
- [ ]
- [ ]
- [ ]

WORKSHEET

Session Reflection

Topics We Covered:	Topics We Did Not Cover:

Likes About My Session:	Dislikes About My Session:

Ah-ha (light bulb) Moments:	Session Reflection:

Homework Assigned:	Topic(s) for Next Session:

My Notes

DATE: ____/____/____

Session Preparation

1. Topics I want to Cover

2. Topics I don't want to Cover

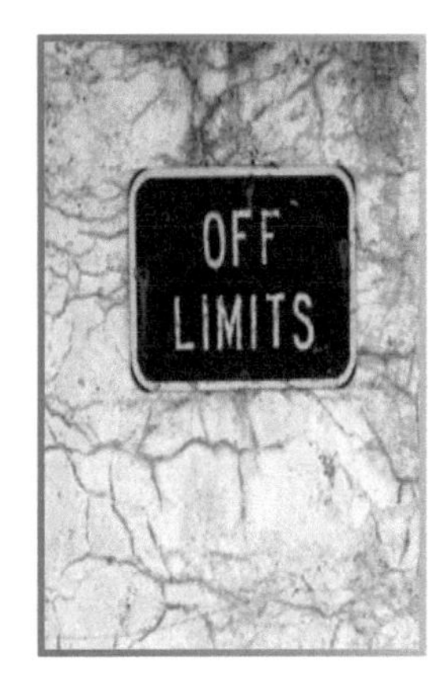

3. Reflections from last session & homework (if applicable)

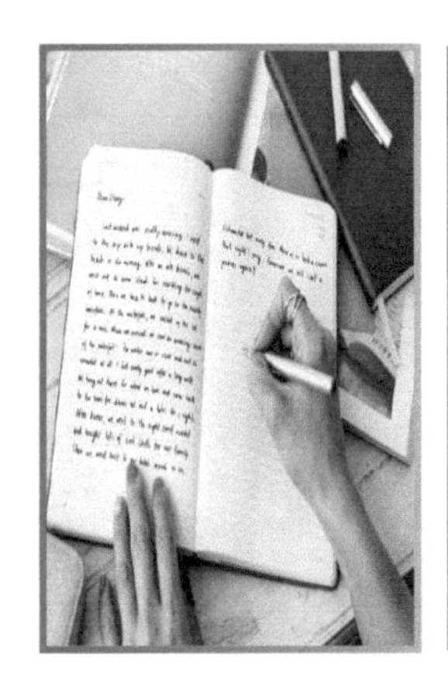

In - Session Notes

DATE: ___/___/___

- [ ]

- [ ]

- [ ]

- [ ]

- [ ]

- [ ]

WORKSHEET

Session Reflection

Topics We Covered:	Topics We Did Not Cover:

Likes About My Session:	Dislikes About My Session:

Ah-ha (light bulb) Moments:	Session Reflection:

Homework Assigned:	Topic(s) for Next Session:

My Notes

DATE: ____/____/____

Session Preparation

1. Topics I want to Cover

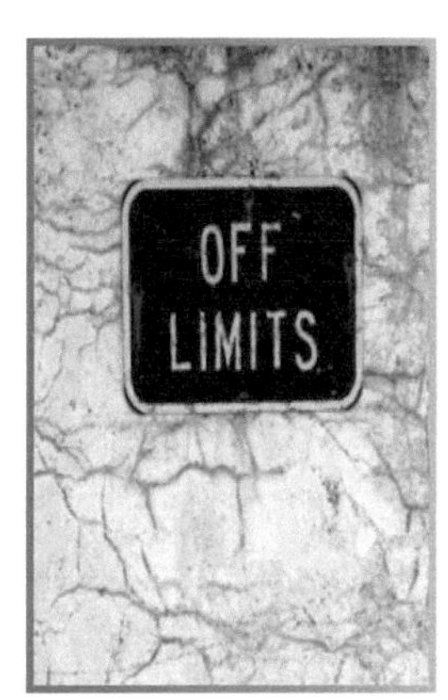

2. Topics I don't want to Cover

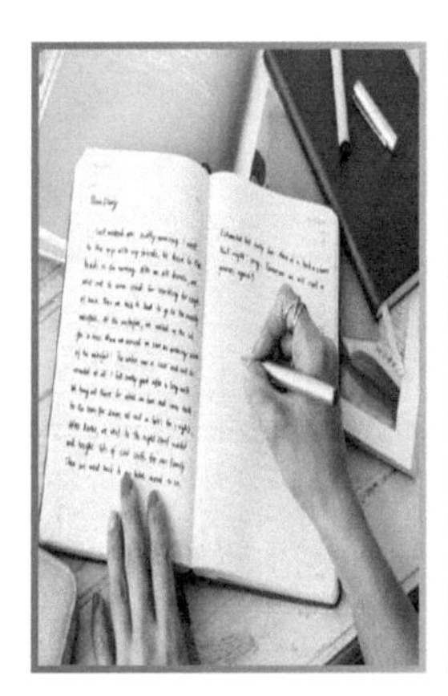

3. Reflections from last session & homework (if applicable)

In - Session Notes

DATE: ___ / ___ / ___

- [ ]
- [ ]
- [ ]
- [ ]
- [ ]
- [ ]

WORKSHEET

Session Reflection

Topics We Covered:	Topics We Did Not Cover:

Likes About My Session:	Dislikes About My Session:

Ah-ha (light bulb) Moments:	Session Reflection:

Homework Assigned:	Topic(s) for Next Session:

My Notes

DATE: ____/____/____

CHECK UP

1-Year ✓

Use this page to assess where you are 1 year into your counseling or coaching process. Share your responses with your counselor or coach, or use the answer stodis cursing your Session Preparation Form.

What Were The Important Sessions of The Month?	Any changes to thoughts?

Any Changes to Emotions/ Feelings?	Any Changes to Behavior?

Am I Where I Was/ Began?	Am I Moving at The Right Pace? Do See Movement?

What I learned ABOUT ME

What Are The Most Important things you learned in coaching or counseling?

What have you learned about the way you see your self,the world, other people, and the future?

What coping strategies and skills have you developed to target your problem areas or goals?

What boundaries do I need to set for people places, and things?

PROCESSING NOTES
What I learned About Me

What are the most important things you learned in coaching or counseling?

What have you learned about the way you see yourself, the world, and the future?

What boundaries do I need to set for people, places, and things?

What coping strategies and skills have you developed to target your problem areas for goals?

Have you noticed any other changes or observations?

Your GUIDED INTERVENTIONS

Activities, Exercises, and Assignments to help you process, learn, and move forward in your healing journey.

Important Note: These activities are exercises created to be used in conjunction with your coach or counselor, or you can complete them on your own. They were created to help you learn more about yourself, behaviors, thoughts, and emotions by utilizing tools that increase self-reflection and cognitive processing. Although you may be tempted to complete multiple worksheets at once, I recommend that you complete them one at a time. Also, allow your self the time to process the results of your activity and possibly discuss them in an upcoming session.

Individual Gardening Activity

The purpose of this activity is for you to think more clearly about the issues you are trying to improve this season. It will allow you to list each one and better understand their importance to you. Following the instructions below will also allow you to understand what is influencing your thoughts and behaviors. Every individual has their own garden for which they're responsible for. You are responsible for your own garden and taking care of its needs. You, in the end, determine the growth, prosperity, and residual (harvest) potential.

Instructions:

1. List what issues you believe belong in your garden.
2. Determine the pros and cons of each item.
3. When difficultly arises when deciding what belongs in which garden, Pray/Meditate, Take a Step Back,and Come Back Later.

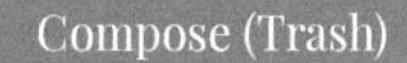

Compose (Trash)

Tips:

1. Be mindful of what you are planting in your garden. = Everything can't be planted at once as too many items can affect the soil and lack growth.
2. Be strategic in where you plant your garden. = Must have proper sunlight to grow, and plants are different in size/height.
3. Use proper tools. Keep tools lubricated to prevent jamming or breaking. = You must tend to your garden & remove weeds, bugs, etc....
4. Keep properly watered & fed. = Water is 2nd key ingredient to growth. Every living organism needs it.
5. Protect plants or move them inside during cold weather. = Too much cold (negative behavior, moods, communication) can cause death in your garden.
6. Rotate plants to sustain the soil. = Rotate every season.

The Miracle Question

The Miracle Question is a goal-setting question that can be helpful when you are dealing with trying to make a decision or you don't know what your future holds. It can also be useful with setting the course for coaching or counseling.

Imagine that tonight, as you sleep, a miracle occurs in your life. Because you were asleep, you didn't know it had happened. When you wake in the morning, how will you be able to tell that the miracle has happened?

Ask Yourself...

- 'What will I see that is different?'
- 'What will I hear that is different?'
- 'What will I be that is different?'
- 'What will I feel inside that is different from the way I feel now?'
- 'What would the other people in my life see, hear, notice that was different?'
- "What would I be like if the miracle has happened, and it magically rid of my problem?"
- "What would I be doing? What could I do that I don't do now?"

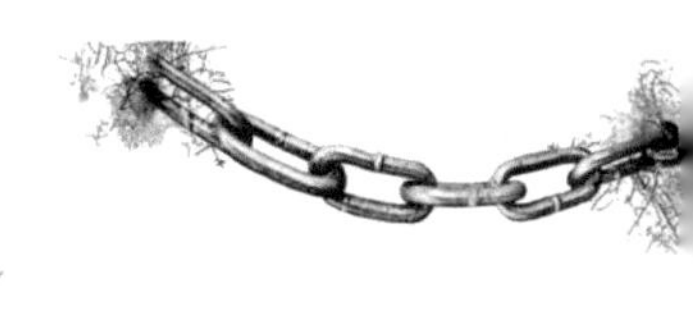

Breaking Chains

When training baby animals in a circus, they often place a chain around the animal's leg and tie them to a pole. Even while tied, the baby animal continues to try to break free, but no matter how hard it tries, it cannot break free. Once fully grown, they now have the strength to break the chain, but by the experience of being tied to a pole, they don't even try. They're unaware of the opportunities and freedomsthat lie ahead.

What Does That Have To Do With Me?

Much like baby animals, we have been "trained" to have negative thoughts about ourselves and difficult events from the past. We have the ability to be free, but we no longer try even when given the opportunity to try. Then list some potential ways you can begin to break every chain.

What are Some Chains (i.e., People, Places, Things or Memories) That are Holding Your Back?

Self Love

In the spaces below, list all the ways you can show love and appreciation to yourself.

Ultimate Coping Playlist

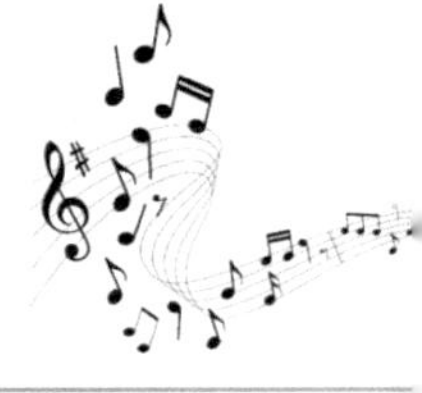

Make the perfect coping playlist for you by giving this challenge a try.

Reminders	A song that reminds you of things you have overcame when you hear it.	A song that reminds you to remain hopeful or optimistic when you hear it.	A song that reminds you of your successes and strengths when you hear it.
Entertainment	A song that stays stuck in your head when you hear it	A song you know all the words to.	Your favorite song from a movie.
Revival	A song that represents freedom	A song that you'd listen to fall asleep.	A song that makes you feel pumped up.
Strong Sensation	A song that reminds you of a good memory.	A song that reminds you of someone you care about	A song that reminds you of someone who cares about you
Diversion	A song that makes you feel safe.	A song you find inspirational.	Your go to positivity song.
Discharge	A song that matches your vibe you get when you feel anxious or worried.	A song that matches your vibe when you feel annoyed or angry.	A song that matches your vibe when you feel sad or afraid.

Resilience Strategies

Write strategies that you have used in the past, or could use in the future to help you successfully over come a challenge.

Grounding Technique

5-4-3-2-1

A calming technique that connects you with the present by exploring the five senses.

Instructions: Sitting or standing, take a deep breath in, and complete the following questions.

5	5 things you can see	
4	4 things you can touch	
3	3 things you can hear	
2	2 things you can smell	
1	1 thing you can taste	

Deep Breathing Exercise

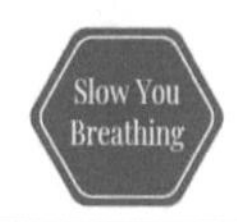

SIT OR LIE DOWN

somewhere comfortable

CLOSE YOUR EYES

helps with limiting distractions

BREATHE IN THROUGH YOUR NOSE

for (4) counts

HOLD YOUR BREATH

for (2) counts

BREATHE OUT THROUGH YOUR NOSE

for (6) counts

REPEAT

practice once or twice a day

Limiting Beliefs

Limiting beliefs and fears can prevent you from achieving goals. This worksheet is used to clear any limiting beliefs you may have that keep you from living your most authentic and best life. Try to identify other beliefs that are holding you back and how you can reframe them to be more productive.

Pick a current issue or belief that would like to clear.

Current Belief	Better Alternatives
Current Belief	Better Alternatives

How has this belief helped or saved you?

Give yourself permission to move on and thank your past beliefs for protecting you.

Is this belief still needed? Is there evidence to support the belief?

I give myself permission to ...

Unhealthy Thinking Styles

All or Nothing Thinking

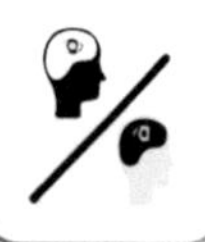

Also called 'black and white thinking'. Things are either all good or all bad.

If I' don't ace every exam, then I am a failure".

Over-Generalizing

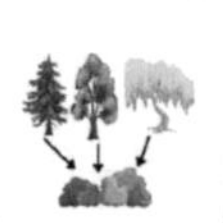

Making a broad generalization about a situation or event based upon a single event.

I always say the wrong things in meetings".

Mental Filter

Having a form of tunnel vision where you only focus on a part of something and don't notice the rest.

"Noticing our failures but not our successes".

Disqualifying the Positive

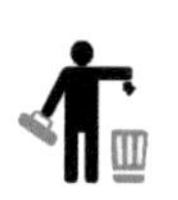

Ignoring the positives whilst focusing only on the negative.

"That doesn't count"...

Jumping to Conclusions

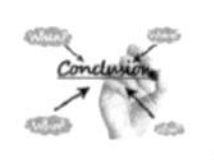

There are two types:
Mind Reading (Assuming you know what other people are thinking.)

Fortune Telling (Believing you can predict what is going to happen.)

Magnification (catastrophizing) & Minimization

Imagining and believing that the worst possible thing will happen, even though the reality is that the problem itself is quite small (catastrophizing), or inappropriately making things seem less important..

Emotional Reasoning

You let your emotions dictate how you perceive a situation.

"I feel stupid, so it must be true".

Should Must

Putting unreasonable demands or pressure on yourself and others.

If we apply 'shoulds' to other people they can create unrealistic expectations.

Labeling

Labeling yourself or other people in certain ways based on behavior in specific situations; despite facts that contradict your labels. I'm not enough... They're so selfish...

Personalization

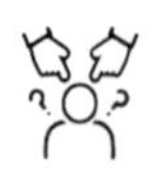

Blaming yourself when things go wrong or could go wrong, even when you may only be partly responsible or not responsible at all. Conversely, blaming other people for things that are your fault.

Thinking Traps Assessment

Rate the questions below on the following scale:

1 = "I never think this way" 2 = "I sometimes think this way" 3 = "I always think this way"

1. ___ I need others to approve of me in order to feel that I am worth something.
2. ___ I feel like a fortune teller, predicting bad things will happen to me.
3. ___ I believe others think about me in a negative way.
4. ___ I tend to discount the good things about me.
5. ___ I either like a person or do not; there is no in-between for me.
6. ___ I minimize the importance of even serious situations.
7. ___ I compare myself to others all the time.
8. ___ I amplify things well beyond their real importance in life.
9. ___ I act as if I have a crystal ball, forecasting negative events in my life.
10. ___What others think about me is more important than what I think about myself.
11. ___ It doesn't matter what my choices are; they always fall flat.
12. ___I make decisions on the basis of my feelings.
13. ___I draw conclusions without carefully reviewing necessary details.
14. ___If a problem develops in my life, you can bet it has something to do with the way I am.
15. ___To feel good, I need others to recognize me.
16. ___I must have things my way in my life.
17. ___I have a tendency to blame myself for bad things.
18. ___Without even asking, I think other people see me in a negative light.
19. ___I do few things as well as others.
20. ___I hold myself responsible for things that are beyond my control.
21. ___I tend not to emphasize the positive traits I have.
22. ___Things seem to go all right or all wrong in my world.
23. ___ I tend to pick out negative details in a situation and dwell on them.

1 = "I never think this way" 2 = "I sometimes think this way" 3 = "I always think this way"

24. ___I have a tendency to exaggerate the importance of minor events.
25. ___I have a habit of predicting that things will go wrong in any given situation.
26. ___I have a lot of should, oughts, and musts in my life.
27. ___I downplay my accomplishments.
28. ___I have been known to make a mountain out of a molehill.
29. ___Most people are better at things than I am.
30. ___When a new rule comes out at school, work, or home, I think it must have been made because of something I did.
31. ___When faced with several possible outcomes, I tend to think the worst is going to happen.
32. ___Things ought to be a certain way.
33. ___If I feel a certain way about something, I am usually right.

Thinking Traps Worksheet

Rate the questions below on the following scale:

1 = "I never think this way" 2 = "I sometimes think this way" 3 = "I always think this way."

34. ___In my mind, things are either black or white; there are no grey areas.
35. ___People only say nice things to me because they want something or because they are trying to flatter me.
36. ___I find I have a tendency to minimize the consequences of my actions, especially if they result in negative outcomes.
37. ___I jump to conclusions without considering alternative points of view.
38. ___If people ignore me, I think they have negative thoughts about me.
39. ___My feelings reflect the way things are.
40. ___When something negative happens, it is just terrible.
41. ___ I tend to dwell on the things I do not like about myself.
42. ___I tend to filter out the positives in a situation and focus more on the negatives.

THINKING TRAPS WORKSHEET

Scoring

Externalization of Self Worth (1, 10, 15)

The development and maintenance of self-worth based almost exclusively on how the external world views you.

Fortune Telling (2, 9, 25) ________

The process of foretelling or predicting the negative outcome of a future event or events and believing this prediction is absolutely true for you.

Mind Reading (3, 18, 38) ________

One's arbitrary conclusion that someone is reacting negatively, or thinking negatively toward him/her, without specific evidence to support that conclusion.

Disqualify the Positive (4, 21, 35) ________

The process of rejecting or discounting positive experiences, traits, or attributes.

Black / White Thinking (5, 22, 34) ________

The tendency to view all experiences as fitting into one of two categories (e.g., positive or negative; good or bad) without the ability to place oneself, others, and experiences along a continuum.

Minimization (6, 27, 36) ________

The process of minimizing or discounting the importance of some event, trait, or circumstance.

Comparison (7, 19, 29) ________

The tendency to compare oneself whereby the outcome typically results in the conclusion that one is inferior or worse off than others.

Magnification (8, 24, 28) ________

The tendency to exaggerate or magnify either the positive or negative importance or consequence of some personal trait, event, or circumstance.

Over-Generalization (11, 14, 40) ________

The process of formulating rules or conclusions based on limited experience and applying theserules across broad and unrelated situations.

Emotional Reasoning (12, 33, 39) ________

The predominant use of an emotional state to form conclusions about oneself, others, or situations.

Jumping to Conclusions (13, 31, 37) ________

Process of drawing a negative conclusion, in the absence of specific evidence to support that conclusion.

Selective Abstractions (23, 41, 42) ________

The process of exclusively focusing on one negative aspect or detail of a situation, magnifying the importance of that detail, thereby casting the whole situation in a negative context.

Should Statements (16, 26, 32) ________

The process of applying personal standards of behavior, standards for other people, or standards about the way the world functions to all situations. Involves the use of words like "should," "ought," and "must."

Personalization (17, 20, 30) ________

The process of assuming personal causality for situations, events, and reactions of others when there is no evidence supporting that conclusion.

THINKING TRAPS WORKSHEET
Writing Prompts

1. We all fall into thinking traps from time to time. What were your top 3 thinking traps?

#1

#2

#3

2. How do you think these thinking traps may inhibit the following:

a. Your performance?

b. Your long-term goals?

c. Your relationships?

3. For each of your top 3 thinking traps – come up with a strategy that will allow you to think more realistically and effectively in the future.

a. Thinking Trap 1

b. Thinking Trap 2

c. Thinking Trap 3

LIST OF GENERIC *Negative and Positive Beliefs*

Negative beliefs

RESPONSIBILITY/ I AM SOMETHING "WRONG"

I don't deserve love.
I am a bad person.
I am terrible.
I am worthless (inadequate).
I am shameful.
I am not lovable.
I am not good enough.
I deserve only bad things.
I am permanently damaged.
I am ugly (my body is hateful).
I do not deserve . . .
I am stupid (not smart enough).
I am insignificant (unimportant).
I am a disappointment.
I deserve to die.
I deserve to be miserable.
I am different (don't belong).

RESPONSIBILITY/ I DID SOMETHING "WRONG"

I should have done something.
I did something wrong.
I should have known better.

SAFETY/ VULNERABILITY

I cannot be trusted.
I cannot trust myself.
I cannot trust my judgment.
I cannot trust anyone.
I cannot protect myself.
I am in danger.
It's not okay to feel (show) my emotions.
I cannot stand up for myself.
I cannot let it out.

CONTROL/ CHOICE

I am not in control.
I am powerless (helpless).
I am weak.
I cannot get what I want.
I am a failure (will fail).
I cannot succeed.
I have to be perfect (please everyone).
I cannot stand it.
I am inadequate.
I cannot trust anyone.

Positive beliefs

I deserve love; I can have love.
I am a good (loving) person.
I am fine as I am.
I am worthy; I am worthwhile.
I am honorable.
I am lovable.
I am deserving (fine/okay).
I deserve good things.
I am (can be) healthy.
I am fine (attractive/ lovable).
I can have (deserve) . . .
I am intelligent (able to learn).
I am significant (important).
I am okay just the way I am.
I deserve to live.
I deserve to be happy.
I am okay as I am.

I did the best I could.
I learned (can learn) from it.
I do the best I can (I can learn).
I can be trusted.
I can (learn to) trust myself.
I can trust my judgment.
I can choose whom to trust.
I can (learn to) take care of myself.
It's over; I am safe now.
I can safely feel (show) my emotions.
I can make my needs known.
I can choose to let it out.

I am now in control.
I do not have choices.
I am strong.
I can get what I want.
I can succeed.
I can succeed.
I can be myself (make mistakes).
I can handle it.
I am capable.
I can choose whom to trust.

CHALLENGING

Unwanted or Anxious Thoughts

Awareness or anxious or unwanted thoughts
Write down the unwanted or anxious thoughts.

What is the current situation?
Where are you, who are you with, and what are you doing?

What is the current situation?
What are you feeling? Where is the feeling or symptom located in your body?

What trap thinking (thought patterns) do you recognize?

Is there evidence to support or go against the thought or belief?

Challenge my anxious thoughts
Change how you are viewing the situation. Have you worried about this problem before? How will worrying or thinking this way help me? How will it hurt me?

Identify solutions to your worries & alternative beliefs

CHALLENGING
Negative Behaviors & Beliefs

Write down the unwanted or anxious thoughts and/or behavior.

Precedent Event/ Trigger(s) (What typically occurs before the negative behavior or thought.)

What does this behavior/ or thought do for you? (How does it protect you?)

Which defense mechanism are you suing? (Fight, Flight, Freeze, Fawn)

Where/Whom did you learn this behavior from?

What is the Root Belief/ Core Belief that you believe about yourself?

Is the behavior or thought still needed to protect you?

What are Some Alternative Behaviors & Beliefs.

NEGATIVE BEHAVIORS & BELIEFS
Impact on Relationships

How have these negative thoughts or behaviors impacted your relationship (s)?

What is your friend, colleague or partner's typical response/ reaction?

Then, how do you react or respond to their words and action?

What plan can you create to stop this cyle? (Do you need tools or resources?)

How will I know that our relationship is improving? (What do you see, hear, feel?)

What is the Root Belief/ Core Belief that you believe about yourself?

Is there any evidence to support this Root/ Core Belief?

FORGIVENESS: I forgive myself for.... I forgive my friend/ spouse/mate for....

DBT House

Creating your house template:

- Draw an outline of the house, including a floor, roof, door, chimney, 4 levels, and a billboard above the house. The house will be used to represent the participant's life. The client can do this, or the therapist can make the template and have the client fill in the rest.

Parts of the house:

- Foundation- On the floor of the house, write the values that govern your life.
- Walls- Along the walls, write anything or anyone who supports you.
- Roof- On the roof, name the things or people that protect you.
- Door- Write the things that you keep hidden from others.
- Chimney- Coming out of the chimney, write down ways in which you blow off steam.
- Billboard- On the billboard, write the things that you are proud of and want others to see.

Levels of the house:

- Level 1: List behaviors that you are trying to gain control of or areas of your life you want to change.
- Level 2: List or draw emotions you want to experience more often, more fully, or in a healthier way.
- Level 3: List all the things you are happy about or want to feel happy about.
- Level 4: List or draw what a "Life Worth Living" would look like for you.

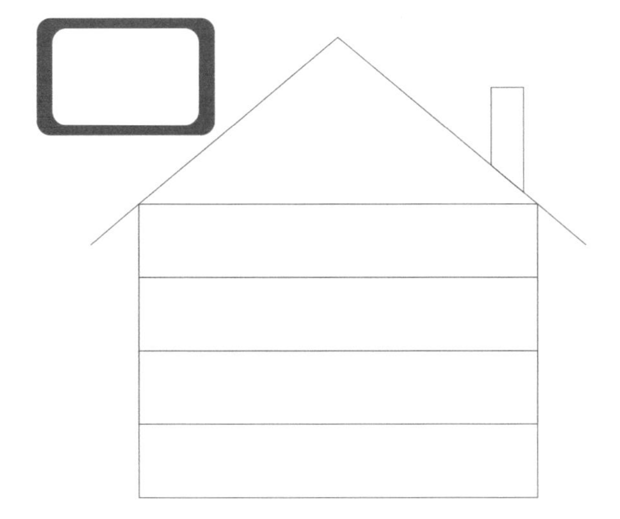

ACTIVITY
The Masks We Wear

Presenting a certain face to the world is something that most people are very familiar with. The different masks that people wear in the course of a day act as a social disguise and help them to get through a variety of situations.

The reasons behind the different masks that people wear vary considerably, but they can be both positive and negative. Some reasons include:

- To gain social acceptance...to be liked
- To hide excitement
- To hide happiness
- To hide vulnerability
- To hide the truth
- To hide fear
- To hide anger
- To hide sadness
- To hide depression
- To hide pain
- To deceive
- To manipulate

We all wear masks at some time in our lives—it's part of human nature. The problem comes when masks become the norm, and we lose ourselves in the process of trying to please others. It is crucial to have selfawareness about the different masks we wear and the reasons behind them-- recognizing the masks we wear is one way to make sure that they do not gain control of our true "self."

> The different masks that people wear can be used positively or negatively. Just be aware you are using them.

ACTIVITY: THE MASKS WE WEAR

Create a mask that shows the different "faces" you present to society. On the LEFT side of the mask, put the faces you show your friends, family, teachers, for example. You can show these behaviors any way you like with pictures, poetry, colors, words/slogans/phrases, etc. On the RIGHT side of the mask, show who you really are. You may have pieces of yourself on the outside of the mask, but you may also have misrepresentations of how people may perceive you. Again, you may illustrate your true self any way you like with pictures, poetry, colors, words/slogans/phrases, etc.

Explain the significance of the images/words/ phrases you chose.

Reflection:

- How difficult is it to be yourself around your family, friends, and other people?
- Who would you find it difficult to be yourself around? Why do you this is true?
- Do you really know who your "self" is?
- What or who influences how you see yourself at any given time?
- How much impact do friends have on how you see yourself? What is the impact of your family, advertising, school, and society?

ACTIVITY
The Masks We Wear

- What are the masks we often wear to hide who we really are?
- How do you feel when you are wearing one of those masks? Phony? Scared? Confident?
- If you were to continue to wear a mask, and you were never allowed to really be yourself,
- What do you think would happen to you over time?
- When was your mask created?
- What does your mask protect you from?
- Is it still needed?

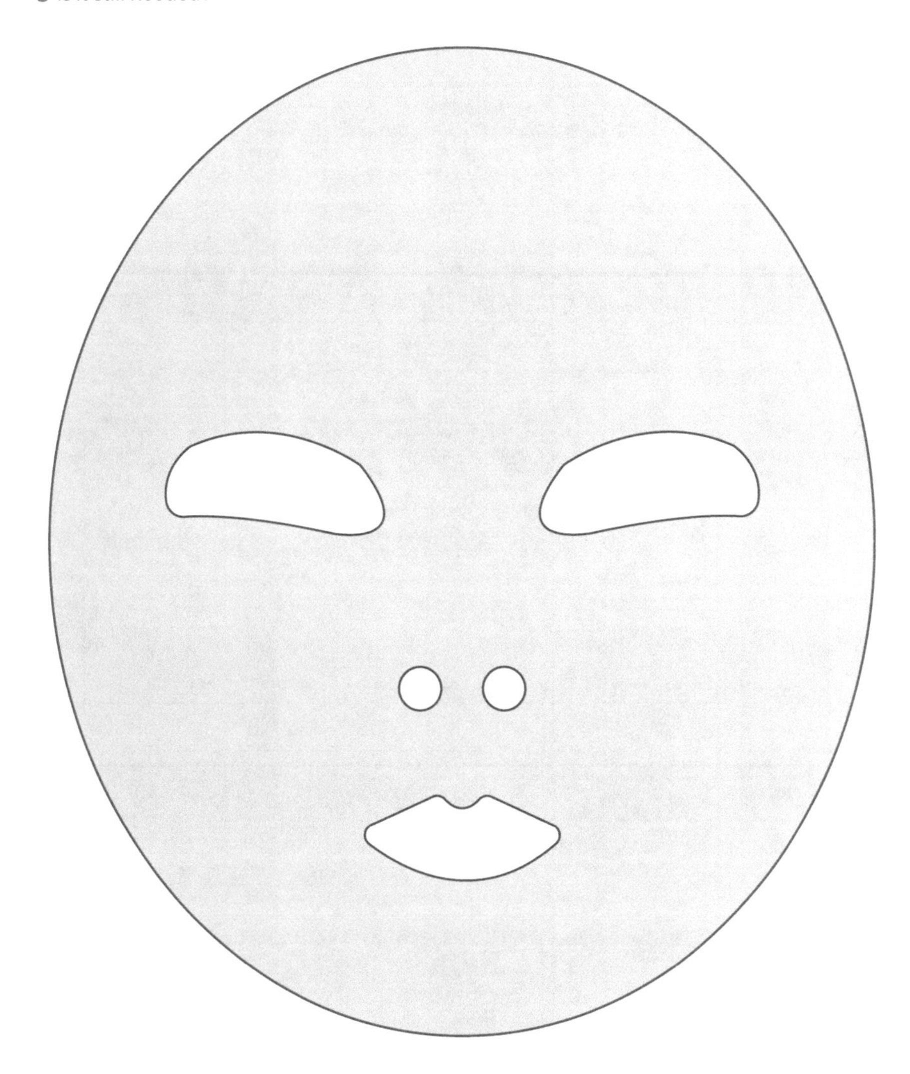

Communicating My Needs

Communicating needs can be hard for some people, whether with family members, relationships, or jobs. This worksheet will use a technique from Dialectal Behavioral Therapy (DBT) called DEAR MAN. This acronym provides step-by-step instructions on developing a strategy to communicate effectively.

Describe the factsof the situation? Don't include opinions

____

Express your feelings using "I" statements: "I feel _____ when_________ ."

____

Assert your self. How will you tell someone what need? What words or language will use?

____

Reinforce you rexpectations. How will you reward the other person for responding well to you?

____

Mindfulness: What is the goal of the interaction? What do you want walkaway knowing feeling?

____

Appear confident by being mindful of your posture and tone of voice and making eye contact.

____

Never accept just anything. What are your limits and non-negotiables?

____

PROMISES, POSSIBILITIES & POTENTIAL: EVALUATING

Unhealthy Relationship Patterns

This worksheet was designed to evaluate patterns of behavior that lead to repeated unhealthy relationships. Though created to focus on romantic relationships, this worksheet can also be modified for family, friends, and peers.

What qualities and contributions do I bring into a relationship?	What qualities or characteristics do I seek in relationships?	What are some unhealthy/toxic qualities seen in current or past relationships?	What are negative core beliefs or roots that tie me to choosing and accepting unhealthy/ toxic qualities in men/ women?	Where/ Whom did you learn this behavior from?	What's my truth? (Positive Affirmation)

Accepting Loss

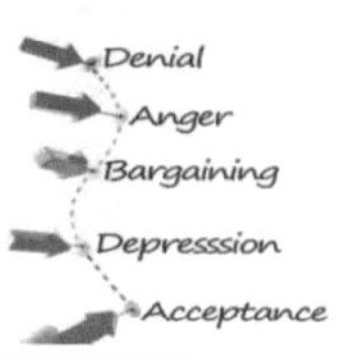

We all face different forms of loss. Loss of jobs, homes, dreams, and even loved ones. It is a natural process that's painful, personal, normal, and unique to each person. How do you process your own loss and begin to create the steps to accept and heal? Creating a process to begin accepting the loss allows a person to come to terms and make sense of their new reality. Use the worksheet below to begin your process.

Accept the reality of the loss. How will you fully accept it, both intellectually and emotionally?

Process and experience the pain of theloss. Know your feelings are valid. List your current feelings.

Adjust to a new reality with what you lost (i.e., Person, place thing). What will life look like daily?

Find a way to remember your loved one and other positive memories. What are some ways to do that?

Watch out for thoughts or behaviors that can derail your healing process. Note any that are present.

Use the tenets of the serenity prayer. What can you accept that you cannot change?

FREE MOBILE APPS
Resources List

Topic	Title & Link	Compatibillity
Addiction Recovery	Recovery Key	iPhone
Anxiety	Stop Panic & Anxiety Self-Help	Android
	Paced Breathing for Managing Anxiety	Android
Depression	QPR	Android
	Positive Activity Jackpot	Android
Eating Disorder Recovery	Recovery Record	iPhone, Android
Focus & Memory	Lumosity Mobile	iPhone
	Time Out Free	iPhone
Meditation	Headspace	iPhone, Android
	Calm	iPhone, Android
	Serenity: Guided Meditation & Mindfulness	iPhone, Android
Mood Tracking & Journaling	Insight Timer	iPhone, Android
	Pacifica - Stress & Anxiety	iPhone, Android
Prescriptions	Mood Tracker by Daylio	iPhone, Android
PTSD	MoodTracker	iPhone, Android
	GoodRx	iPhone, Android
Relationships	PTSD Coach	iPhone, Android
	ptsd.va.gov/appvid/mobile/index.asp	
Sleep	td411	iPhone, Android
	Build Stronger Relationships	Android
	Sleep as Android: Sleep Cycle Alarm	Android
	Fabulous - Motivate Me	Android
	Insight Timer	iPhone, Android
Social Life	Sleep Bot Tracker Log	Android
Stress	Smart Alarm Clock	iPhone
	Meetup	Android
	T2 Mood Tracker	iPhone, Android
	Breathe2Relax	iPhone, Android
	The Worry Box	Android
	EFT Clinic	iPhone
Wellbeing	GPS for the Soul	iPhone
	Happify	iPhone
Women's Health	Five Ways to Wellbeing	Android
	VOS - Wellbeing	iPhone, Android
Decreasing Social Media Use	Clue Period Tracker	iPhone, Android
	Women's Health Tracker	Android
	Offtime	iPhone, Android
	BreakFree	iPhone, Android
	Flipd	iPhone, Android
	AppDetox	Android
	Stay on Task	Android

Congratulations

YOU M A D E IT !!!

While we have reached the final destination in your journal, I hope you will continue on your counseling or coaching journey. Your courage and openness to document the start of your healing or exploratory process will undoubtedly allow you to track your progress and strengthen your knowledge about yourself. By now, I hope you have gained a new appreciation and understanding for your gifts and strengths—a better understanding of your past, beliefs, and values. Even more, you have learned ways to embrace your whole self, including your flaws and imperfections (that we all have), while releasing self-doubt. You may also have found that your relationships and interactions with others have changed. This outcome is perfectly normal and okay. With your coaching or counseling sessions, you have learned new ways to cope, thrive, heal and motivate yourself towards your goals. It is here in this workbook that you can observe how all of the hard work paid off.

Throughout this journey, you may have encountered several high and low moments. You may have even experienced Aha moments -- moments of sudden realization, inspiration, insight, or recognition, or understanding -- surrounding certain memories, events, feelings, or topics. Even through these moments, you didn't give up, and you continued on your healing or exploratory journey. Remember, this is an ongoing journey that continues to evolve daily—so just keep moving forward.

I encourage you to check out the interventions section at the end of this book. Many helpful worksheets are provided that can be utilized in your counseling and coaching sessions or on your own. I feel honored to have created a journal to help you document your navigation to a better you. I wish you all the best on your continued journey.

HOW TO UNDERSTAND COMMON *Counseling Acronyms*

Here's a brief guide to some of the common words and credentials in mental health licensing in the United States. Some of these credentials relate to the state licensing and certification standards for practicing professionals. They do vary from state to state.

- "A" - Associate-level therapists. The clinician is under supervision due to the current completion of mandated hours. Cannot work independently.
- LCSW/LMSW: Licensed Clinical Social Worker/ Licensed Master Social Worker
- LPC/LCPC/LPCC/LMHC: These acronyms stand for, respectively, licensed professional counselor, licensed professional clinical counselor, licensed professional clinical counselor, and licensed mental health counselor.
- LAC/LCAS: In some states, a licensed (clinical) addiction counselor has been licensed as an addictions counselor and has specialized training in this substance use field.
- NCC: A national certified counselor has completed a master's degree, post-degree supervision, and the national counselor examination. This is a nationwide credential.
- LMFT: This stands for licensed marriage and family therapist.
- PsyD: This means the holder has completed a doctorate in psychology degree.
- LP: Some licensed psychologists use this credential to indicate their status. But it is not standard, so many others do not. The only clinicians may offer psychological testing and assessment services. Psychiatric Mental Health.
- Practitioner: (PMHNP) is an advanced practice registered nurse trained to provide a wide range of mental health services (i.e., diagnose, conduct therapy, and prescribe medications for psychiatric disorders or substance abuse problems).
- Psychiatrist: A psychiatrist is a medical doctor (MD) who completed specialized training in the diagnosis and treatment of mental illness.

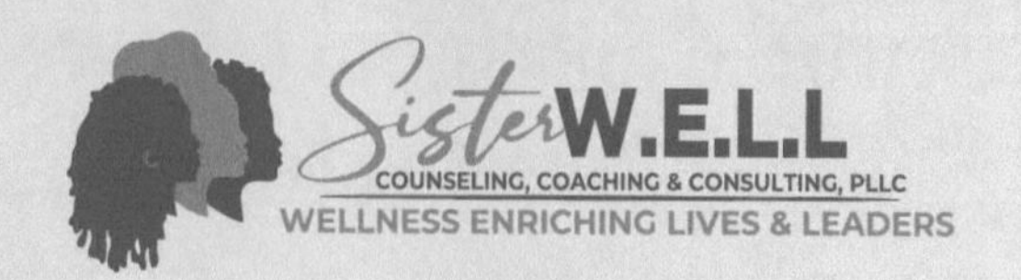

ACKNOWLEDGMENTS

Throughout my life, I have been fortunate to have been surrounded by family, friends, mentors, and colleagues who have encouraged me never to give up and to follow my dreams. Most importantly, to always show up as my authentic self. No matter what it "sounded" like. Thank you, Dr. Shari Sias!

This journal is a culmination of worksheets, exercises, and activities that I have created and used with my clients over the past few years. Something truly sacred and profound happens in a counseling session while holding space for someone to share such vulnerability. It is in these moments that I feel honored, for my clients are the real teachers and healers. They just allow me to walk their journey with them.

I am forever indebted to my husband, Lorinza, for his unwavering support and empowerment throughout this journey. He continued to remind me of my gifts and what I had to share with others. I would also be remiss if I didn't thank my business partners and friends, Dr. Shawnte' Elbert (my identical twin) and Dr. Charla Blumell of Sister WELLS Counseling, Coaching & Consulting. I am also grateful for my children, William and Bryson, Mom, and friends, who have been loving cheerleaders throughout this endeavor.

Finally, a big thank you to my clients who allow me to witness their inspirational courage and dedication as they improve their emotional health and overall well-being. I am genuinely and forever grateful for allowing me to walk this journey with you.

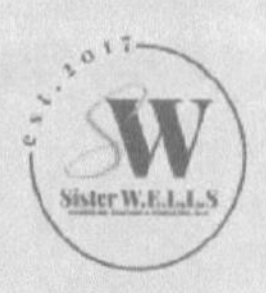

About The Author

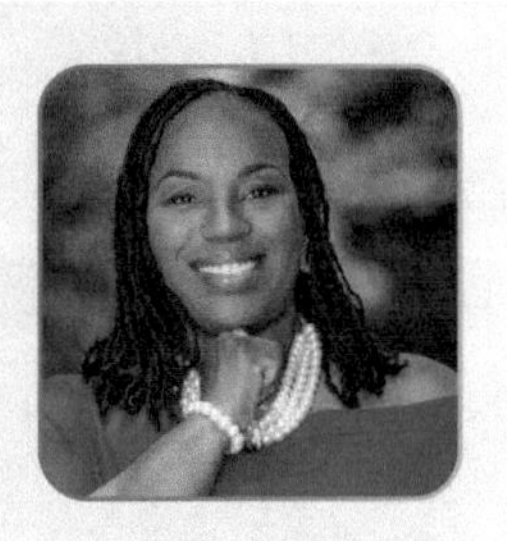

Dr. Sherra' Watkins, Ph.D. is a certified clinical psychotherapist and coach with over 10 years of experience helping her clients overcome a wide range of psychological and emotional issues. With a background in mental health counseling, rehabilitation and addiction recovery, and sexual assault advocacy, Dr. Watkins is passionate about empowering people of all backgrounds to improve their wellbeing and practice emotional healing.

She currently serves as the Director of Wellness Counseling and Assistant Professor in the Department of Behavioral Sciences at American University of the Caribbean School of Medicine in Sint Maarten. A leader in the mental health and substance use field, her passion is to transform systems that perpetuate decreased access and utilization of counseling and addiction services to marginalized populations. As a highly sought-after presenter and keynote speaker, as well as the author of Healing – In Review, she's dedicated to sharing the tools and knowledge her readers need to live happier, healthier, and more fulfilling lives. Dr. Watkins currently resides in Sint Maarten with her husband, Lorinza, and two boys, William and Bryson. For more information, visit www.sisterwells.org.

info@sisterwells.org

@sisterwell

@sisterwells_counseling coaching

Dr. Sherrá Watkins

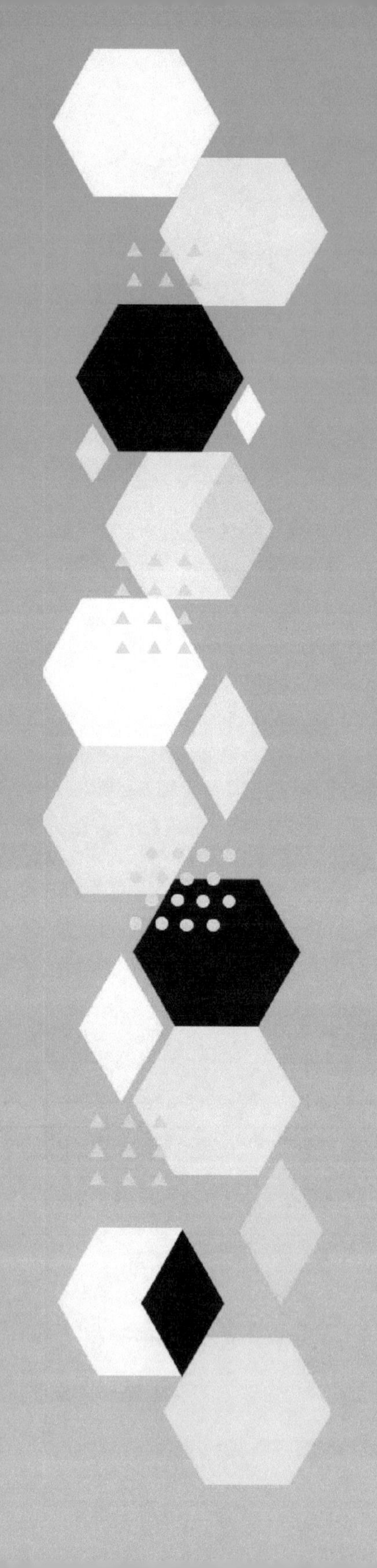

Thanks

For Your Support

Made in United States
Troutdale, OR
09/27/2024